Atlas of Neonatal Histopathology

AUGUSTO MORAGAS

Chief, Department of Pathologic Anatomy,
Barcelona Social Security Health Center;
Professor of Pathologic Anatomy, Faculty
of Medicine, Autonomous University of Barcelona

ANGEL BALLABRIGA

Director, Pediatric Clinic, Barcelona
Social Security Health Center;
Professor of Pediatrics, Faculty of Medicine,
Autonomous University of Barcelona

MARIA TERESA VIDAL

Chief, Section of Pathologic Anatomy,
Barcelona Social Security Health Center;
Associate Professor of Medicine, Faculty of
Medicine, Autonomous University of Barcelona

Translated by

ANTONIO VALDES-DAPENA, M.D.

Clinical Professor of Pathology, University of Miami
School of Medicine, Miami, Florida; Pathologist,
Palm Springs General Hospital, Hialeah, Florida;
Former Director of Pathology, Graduate Hospital,
University of Pennsylvania, Philadelphia, Pennsylvania

MARIE A. VALDES-DAPENA, M.D.

Professor of Pathology and Professor of Pediatrics,
University of Miami School of Medicine, Miami, Florida;
Director, Section of Pediatric Pathology,
Jackson Memorial Hospital, Miami, Florida

1977

W. B. SAUNDERS COMPANY Philadelphia / London / Toronto

W. B. Saunders Company: West Washington Square
Philadelphia, PA   19105

1 St. Anne's Road
Eastbourne, East Sussex BN21 3UN, England

1 Goldthorne Avenue
Toronto, Ontario M8Z 5T9, Canada

Library of Congress Cataloging in Publication Data

Moragas, Augusto.

Atlas of neonatal histopathology.

Translation of Atlas de histopathología neonatal.

Includes index.

1. Infants (Newborn) — Diseases — Atlases.   2. Pediatric
pathology — Atlases.   3. Histology, Pathological —
Atlases.   I. Ballabriga Aguado, Angel, joint author.
II. Vidal, Maria Teresa, joint author.   III. Title.

RJ255.M6713   611'.018   76–45960

ISBN 0–7216–6542–X

Atlas of Neonatal Histopathology   ISBN   0-7216-6542-X

Translation and Adaptation of the first Spanish language edition.
Copyright © 1974 by Salvat Editores, S. A., Mallorca, 41, Barcelona (España)

Last digit is the print number: 9   8   7   6   5   4   3   2   1

Preface

This atlas is based on our experience in neonatal pathology at the Children's Hospital, in the Department of Pathologic Anatomy of the Barcelona Social Security Health Center, and in the School of Medicine of the Autonomous University of Barcelona.

The material upon which this study is based was derived during the last seven years from more than 3,000 autopsies involving infants less than 30 days of age.

We have not only emphasized the histopathologic aspects of each case but have dealt also with clinical and gross anatomical correlations, thus reflecting our conviction that all three must be considered together. Just as clinicians should know and appreciate the importance of the underlying anatomical changes of various diseases, the pathologist must go beyond morphologic alterations to embrace in his study of any case the essential clinical features as well.

In order to set some limits on the length of this work, the authors have decided not to include descriptions of specific gross pathologic changes and to omit many details of the more complex congenital malformations, especially those of the heart and of the genitourinary tract.

In summary, this is an atlas of neonatal histopathology with particular emphasis on clinicoanatomical correlation, prepared for general pathologists, who are frequently confronted with difficult problems in the interpretation of lesions unique to the neonatal period, and for pediatricians in the hope that it will enhance their understanding of the clinical aspects of neonatal disease by virtue of more complete comprehension of the pathologic lesions involved.

Translators' Foreword

The task of translating this very complete and beautifully illustrated piece of work was undertaken by two pathologists together, by one of us because his native language is Spanish and by the other because, in addition to being conversant with that language, she is a pediatric pathologist.

The translation is faithful to the original in every possible respect. Occasionally, on account of the idiosyncrasies of syntax peculiar to every language, the order of words or phrases may have been changed. Likewise, the translation of certain medical terms is not always literal, but the meaning has been preserved.

It must be added that the experience of translating a work based on such extensive material has been highly interesting and most instructive, particularly for the one of us who is not versed in pediatric pathology. It is unquestionable that this atlas will be of tremendous use and interest to the general pathologist who is occasionally confronted with the very special problems of infant pathology as well as to those who cultivate the subspecialty.

ANTONIO M. VALDES-DAPENA, M.D.
MARIE A. VALDES-DAPENA, M.D.

Contents

Index
of Illustrations

RESPIRATORY SYSTEM

HEART

CENTRAL NERVOUS SYSTEM

KIDNEY

ADRENAL GLANDS

THYROID

GENITALIA

LYMPHATIC SYSTEM

THE EYE

SKELETAL SYSTEM

CONGENITAL TUMORS*

*Observed in the first 30 days of life.

Respiratory System

1
PULMONARY IMMATURITY, MINIMAL

Male weighing 1,100 gm at birth. Gestational age, 33 weeks. Apgar score 4 at birth.

Admitted within an hour of birth with decreased muscle tone and cyanosis, and in generally poor condition. pH 7.24, pCO_2 49 mm Hg, BE —9.5 mEq/L, hematocrit 52 per cent. Acidosis corrected by infusion of 10 per cent dextrose and 1 M bicarbonate solution. At 24 hours of life the patient experienced a crisis of apnea and cyanosis, requiring resuscitation. Death ensued 6 hours later.

Histopathologic Study. Lungs: In Figure 1 there is persistence of some tubular structures with cuboidal epithelial lining. Alveolar spaces, however, are predominant. The intimate relationship of capillaries and epithelial alveolar lining cells should be pointed out (H & E, 375×).

Autopsy showed intraventricular and subtentorial cerebral hemorrhage.

At times it is difficult to evaluate apparent collapse of the lung and to distinguish areas of "anectasia" (primary atelectasis, or persistent lack of aeration) from areas of secondary collapse (secondary atelectasis) in portions of lung never previously expanded. An important criterion in adequately fixed material is the persistence of clusters of cuboidal epithelial lining cells (a primitive pattern) with relatively clear and abundant cytoplasm, and rounded nuclei with loose chromatin network. Nonaerated areas (because of primary or secondary atelectasis) may persist for several days, particularly in premature infants. It should also be kept in mind that the alveoli of the mature lung before the onset of respiration are not empty, but are occupied by amniotic fluid formed by the lung rather than aspirated from the amniotic cavity.

2
PULMONARY IMMATURITY, MODERATE

Male, 770 gm in weight. Gestational age, 29 weeks. Apgar score 1 at birth. Resuscitation was required. Cyanosis ensued. Death occurred at 5 hours of life.

Histopathologic Examination. The immaturity of this lung is apparent in the persistence of abundant loose connective tissue stroma, in the midst of which there are rudimentary alveolar ducts, tubular in shape and lined by cuboidal epithelial cells. There is scanty capillary penetration. The capillaries in the intersti-

tial tissue show dilated lumina filled with erythrocytes (H & E, 375×).

3
PULMONARY IMMATURITY, MARKED

Five hundred and fifty gram male. Gestational age, 26 weeks. Breech delivery. Died en route to the hospital.

Histopathologic Examination. The pulmonary parenchyma has a compact appearance, with numerous acinar formations lined by tall epithelium with apparent absence of alveolar differentiation. Vascularization of the parenchyma is reduced to sparse capillaries far removed from the tubular ducts. This picture represents the most marked degree of pulmonary immaturity in our series of infants born alive and surviving a few hours (H & E, 375×).

4
UNILATERAL PULMONARY HYPOPLASIA. LEFT DIAPHRAGMATIC HERNIA

Full-term male weighing 3,000 gm. Vertex delivery. Six hours of labor. Apgar score 1 at 1 minute, necessitating vigorous resuscitation with intubation.

Admitted at 30 minutes of life in moribund condition with loss of muscular tone, pallor, and scaphoid abdomen. Bradycardia was marked. Heart sounds were heard in right hemithorax at level of nipple line; breath sounds were absent over left hemithorax.

Chest x-ray showed translucent areas on the left, with density in the right hemithorax suggesting a large left diaphragmatic hernia and severe lack of pulmonary expansion or hypoplasia of the left lung. Mixed acidosis, both metabolic and respiratory, was ascertained. An infusion of 1 M bicarbonate was given by vein, and it was decided to intervene surgically as an emergency. The infant died at the beginning of the procedure.

Histopathologic Examination. Figure 4 represents a section of the left lung. The close proximity of the pleural surface and relatively large bronchi is conspicuous. The bronchial walls exhibit heavy plaques of hyaline cartilage. The pulmonary parenchyma is atelectatic. In our series of diaphragmatic hernias, marked pulmonary hypoplasia on the same side is usually associated with a certain degree of hypoplasia of the opposite lung. (H & E, 60×)

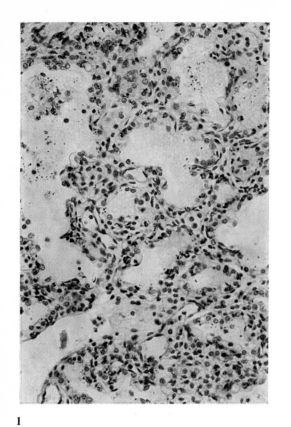

1

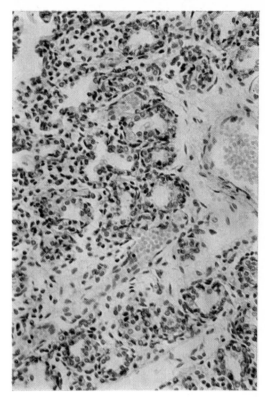

2

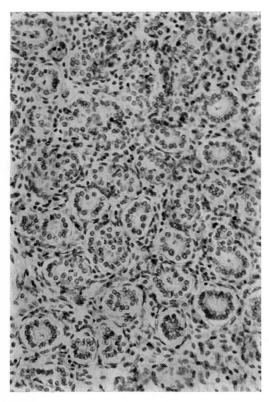

3

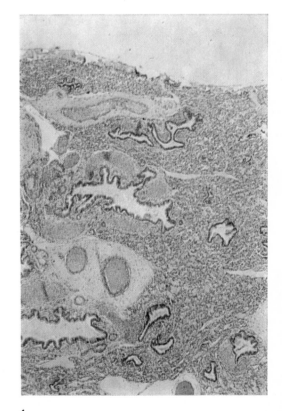

4

5
ASPIRATION OF MECONIUM

Eight hundred and ninety gram female, unknown gestational age. Normal delivery; resuscitation required at birth because of an Apgar score of 1. History of fetal distress during delivery.

Admitted at 30 minutes of life in poor general condition; appearance of marked immaturity, generalized loss of muscle tone, lack of spontaneous motion, generalized cyanosis, and gasping respiration. Placed in an incubator with 100 per cent oxygen. Cyanosis gradually decreased; some spontaneous movements appeared and respiration was established. One half hour later cyanosis reappeared, was followed by an apneic crisis, and the infant died in spite of attempts at resuscitation.

Histopathologic Examination. Figure 5 shows massive filling of air spaces, predominantly by masses of meconium or simply amorphous brownish material. Note the scarcity of keratinized squames. There was moderate pulmonary immaturity with peribronchial emphysema, probably secondary to resuscitation, and there were foci of granulocytic exudate surrounding the aspirated material (H & E, 600×).

Other autopsy findings were: generalized signs of immaturity, petechiae on the lateral aspect of each ventricle, interstitial hemorrhage in the left choroid plexus, and notable narrowing of the colon, with an empty lumen as a sign of fetal distress. There was also dilatation of the right atrium.

Aspiration of meconium or amniotic fluid or both is infrequent in infants early in gestation and is usually observed in newborns near term. In our series of 120 cases of amniotic fluid and meconium aspiration, only 30 per cent were infants with body weights less than 2,500 gm.

Lesions that are commonly observed in infants with massive meconium or amniotic fluid aspiration are the presence of areas of excessive expansion of the lung (presumably either compensatory or the result of efforts at resuscitation) alternating with areas of resorptive atelectasis.

6/7/8
MASSIVE ASPIRATION OF AMNIOTIC DEBRIS

Male infant born at term weighing 3,600 gm. Signs of fetal distress during delivery. Breech presentation. No spontaneous cry. Apgar score 4. Irregular, superficial respiration. Progressive increase of respiratory rate. At 4 hours, a prolonged apneic episode forced attempts at resuscitation. Bicarbonate solution was given to correct the acidosis. Death occurred at 6 hours.

Histopathologic Examination. Many bronchioles presented the appearance shown in Figure 6: a dilated lumen filled with a large number of squamous epithelial cells (H & E, 375×). The aspirated material reached the most distal portions of the respiratory tree. Figure 7 shows the alveolar lumina to be filled and distended with squamous cells with eosinophilic cytoplasm and pyknotic nuclei (H & E, 600×). In Figure 8 the aspiration of squames is associated with the presence of abundant PAS-positive mucoid material. It is also associated with the presence of a certain number of polymorphonuclear leukocytes (375×).

The presence of large numbers of squamous cells in the lungs of a newborn is a clue to the prior occurrence of intrauterine anoxic episodes, which presumably induced gasping respiration. On the other hand, their *absence* does not exclude intrauterine anoxia, inasmuch as the amniotic debris can be expelled after being aspirated or there may not have been any aspiration because death occurred so rapidly or because the nasal and buccal orifices of the fetus were occluded.

In our experience there is usually no relationship between excessive aspiration of amniotic debris and intrauterine pneumonia. In those cases in which both lesions coexist the involvement usually affects different portions of the lung; there is no correlation between the two processes, either in extent or in intensity. In this case there was subpleural vesicular emphysema with hydrothorax accompanied by pericardial effusion and punctate intracerebral hemorrhages of an anoxic type.

Small groups of intraalveolar squamous cells may be encountered in the lungs of older infants, even at a month and a half of age; they seem to have no pathologic significance.

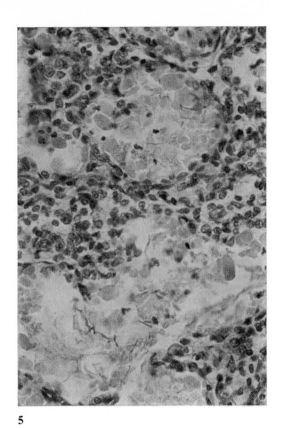

5

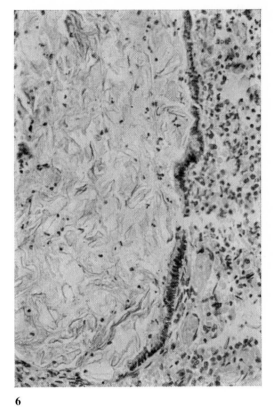

6

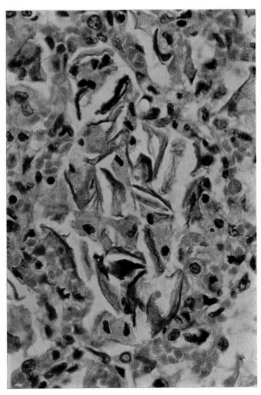

7

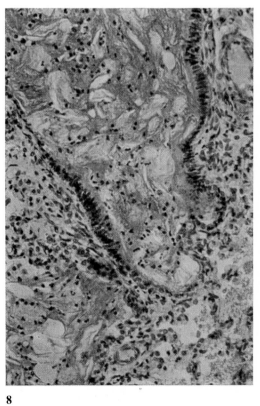

8

PNEUMONIA DUE TO ASPIRATION OF GASTRIC CONTENTS

Female weighing 1,100 gm. Gestational age, 32 weeks. Breech presentation. Apgar score 6.

Admitted 20 minutes after birth in poor general condition with signs of immaturity and loss of muscle tone.

The infant was placed in an incubator and given a slow infusion of 10 per cent dextrose. No feedings were administered. Signs of respiratory insufficiency continued. Twenty-four hours later there was an episode of apnea and cyanosis. Efforts at resuscitation failed.

Histopathologic Examination. Both lungs, but particularly the right upper lobe, showed multiple small irregular necrotic foci filled with microorganisms and surrounded by moderate polymorphonuclear infiltration. This was especially marked in the more peripheral portions of the lungs (Fig. 9, H & E, 60×). In places it was possible to see the aspirated material occupying the lumina of bronchioles. There was also macrophage infiltration.

In other more recent foci, seen in Figure 10, there was only necrobiosis with destruction of the alveolar septa, which are identifiable as architectural shadows, with occasional pyknotic nuclei. This area was filled with a light eosinophilic fluid, rich in microorganisms. The wall of the adjacent bronchiole is partially destroyed but shows no inflammatory reaction (H & E, 375×).

Other lesions demonstrated at autopsy in this case included the presence of cytomegaly in the adrenal, marked atrophy of the thymus, and subarachnoid microcysts.

It must be remembered that isolated patterns similar to those illustrated in Figure 10 can be explained on the basis of postmortem autolysis as a result of the aspiration of gastric contents. Similarly, areas of necrosis like those shown here may be seen in the course of *Pseudomonas* sepsis; in such cases there are usually areas of necrosis in other organs. An important differential characteristic is the fact that, in true aspiration, the necrotic zone includes a bronchus or bronchiole at its center, whereas in the septic necrotic foci of *Pseudomonas* infection, there is usually a blood vessel at the center with necrotic walls and abundant microorganisms. In the lung these septic "foci" show a special preference for peribronchial vessels.

ASPIRATION OF BILE-STAINED MATERIAL

Newborn at term, male, weighing 2,950 gm. Admitted at 3 days of age because of a 24 hour episode of expiratory wheezing, signs of respiratory insufficiency, refusal to feed, absence of spontaneous bowel movements, deep jaundice, generalized loss of muscle tone, and purulent vesicles about the neck. On admission, while an intravenous infusion was being attempted, the infant suddenly vomited bright red blood and died.

Histopathologic Examination. The autopsy showed evidence of a septic process. The liver exhibited bile stasis with necrotizing granulomas. Similar foci were demonstrable in the adrenals, which also showed thrombi in medullary vessels. The lungs showed bronchopneumonia; a number of terminal bronchioles were lined by a layer of finely lumpy golden-yellow material (Fig. 11, H & E, 375×). In this illustration erythrocytes are seen in some of the alveoli, as well as a small number of squamous cells. This yellowish material was most conspicuous in the subpleural portions of the lung, where it occupied most of the alveolar spaces. The lighter band at the bottom of the illustration represents subpleural connective tissue (Fig. 12, H & E, 375×).

The absence of pigmentation in the portions of the lung with pneumonia suggests the possibility of inhalation of bile in vomitus rather than bile staining of an exudate produced by some other mechanism. As there is no inflammatory reaction to the pigment, its deposition may be a terminal phenomenon.

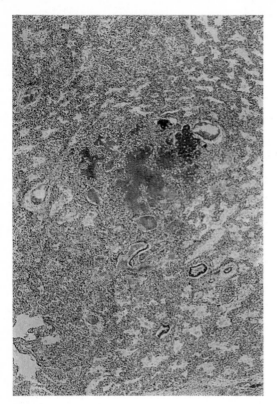

9

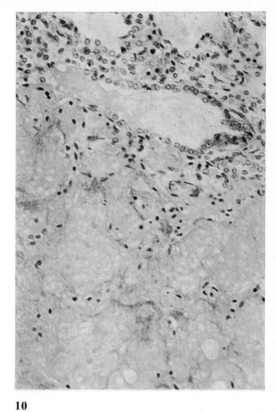

10

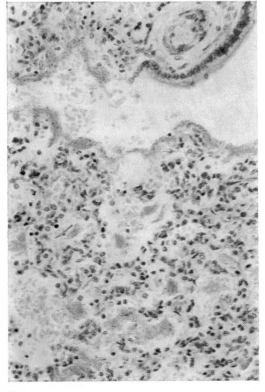

11

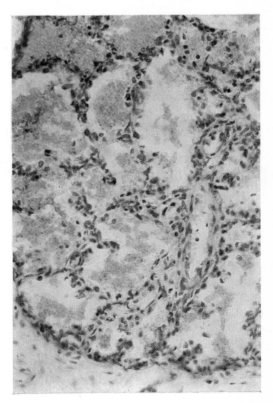

12

13/14
INTRAUTERINE PNEUMONIA

Five hundred and ninety gram female with gestational age of 25 weeks. Apgar score 2 at birth.

The infant was admitted at 1 hour of age with gasping respiration, generalized cyanosis, complete loss of muscle tone, and edema of the extremities.

Death occurred 1 hour later.

Histopathologic Examination. Figure 13 depicts intrauterine pneumonia associated with pulmonary immaturity; more often than not this is seen in the prematurely born. Granulocytic exudate is diffuse and affects most of the lung. In this illustration pulmonary immaturity is evident in the tubular character of the air spaces, which are lined by cuboidal epithelium. There are no visible alveoli. Furthermore, the air spaces are separated from one another by abundant loose connective tissue stroma with capillaries that are relatively far from the air-bearing lumina. Many of the air spaces are completely filled with polymorphonuclear leukocytes. There is no fibrin in the exudate, and there is no septal necrosis (H & E, 375×).

In our experience, in a total of 1,364 neonatal autopsies, we have observed this type of pneumonia in 10.83 per cent of prematures and in 9.88 per cent of full-term newborns dying during the first day of life. In the subsequent 24 hour period this percentage increased slightly in prematures (13.64 per cent) but did not change appreciably among full-term infants (9.3 per cent). In the third day of life, the number of cases of intrauterine pneumonia decreased visibly in both groups to values to below 4 per cent.

It is interesting to note that in all infants dying of intrauterine pneumonia during the first 24 hours of life (55 cases) the incidence varied considerably depending on the weight of the infant. Thus, in prematures weighing less than 1,000 gm the incidence was 40 per cent of the total; in the group between 1,000 and 1,500 gm it was 12.8 per cent; between 1,501 and 2,000 gm, 7.3 per cent; between 2,001 and 2,500, 10.9 per cent; between 2,501 and 3,000, 9.1 per cent; from 3,001 to 3,500 gm, 7.3 per cent; and

in those with weights above 3,500 gm it was 12.7 per cent. In full-term newborns intrauterine pneumonia was usually associated with premature rupture of the membranes and prolonged or difficult labor. Figure 14 illustrates intrauterine pneumonia in a male infant born at term (H & E, 375×).

15/16
INTRAUTERINE PNEUMONIA WITH GIANT CELLS

Nine hundred and fifty gram male, gestational age, 28 weeks. Vertex presentation. Artificial rupture of membranes 15 minutes before delivery. Duration of labor, 3 hours. Maternal history, three abortions.

Admitted at 15 minutes of age.

Loss of muscle tone. Cyanosis, bradycardia. Reflexes absent. Death 2 hours after admission. No history of recent measles or rubella in the mother.

Histopathologic Examination. The alveolar spaces are occupied by a granulocytic exudate with some mononuclear cells. In some fields there are giant cells with multiple nuclei, abundant cytoplasm, and some vacuoles but without signs of any foreign material or inclusion bodies (Fig. 15, H & E, 375×). Nevertheless, in an occasional microscopic field, globular hyaline masses containing nuclear remnants can be observed (Fig. 16, H & E, 375×).

There was no hemorrhagic infiltration. The postpartum survival of less than 3 hours suggests that the process had an intrauterine origin.

This picture should not be confused with the so-called interstitial giant cell pneumonia attributable to measles virus and observable in later periods of life. In those cases, giant cells with intranuclear cytoplasmic inclusions are seen as well as lesions characterized by interstitial round cell infiltration, swelling of the alveolar cells, hyaline membranes, and abundant squamous metaplasia of the lining of bronchioles. Pneumonia with the presence of giant cells as a reaction to foreign material can be seen in Figures 55 and 56.

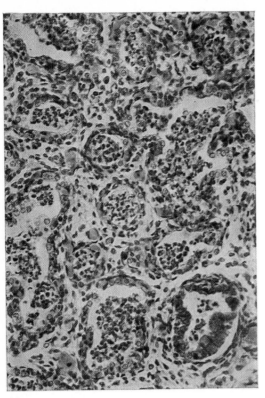

13

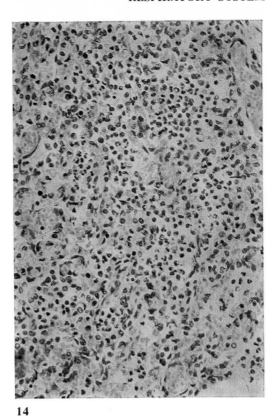

14

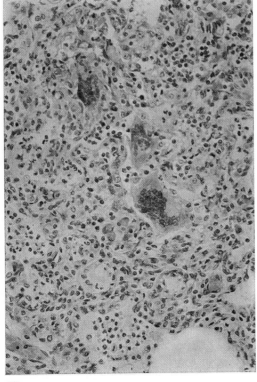

15

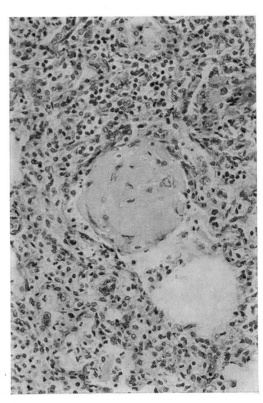

16

17/18
PNEUMONIA ACQUIRED IN UTERO

Female weighing 2,200 gm of unknown gestational age. Labor of 3 hours' duration. Rupture of membranes 4 days before delivery. At birth, spontaneous cry was absent and there was gasping respiration. She was admitted at 30 minutes of life. Poor general state. Cyanosis. Loss of muscle tone. X-ray of the chest at 4 hours showed diffuse finely nodular densities in both lung fields. Death occurred at 22 hours in a picture of progressive respiratory insufficiency. pH 7.07, pCO_2 78 mm Hg, BE -11 mEq/L. Blood culture was obtained by catheterization of the umbilical artery and was positive for *Pneumococcus*. Culture of aspirated gastric contents was positive for *Pneumococcus*. Meconium and urine cultures were negative. Smears of umbilical cord were negative.

Histopathologic Examination. In spite of a survival of only 22 hours the findings on histologic examination are those of bronchopneumonia acquired postnatally, a uniform, diffuse granulocytic pneumonia with fibrin and grampositive cocci.

Figure 17 shows the massive character of the inflammatory exudate with a great quantity of polymorphonuclear leukocytes in the alveolar spaces and marked septal congestion. In the center of the lower portion of the picture, an intensely acidophilic band is observed attached to the lining of an alveolar duct. It has the characteristics of a hyaline membrane (H & E, 187.5×).

In other fields and with greater magnification, the presence of extensive networks of fibrin can be observed, extending freely from one air space to another. In these areas erythrocytes are noted among the meshes of fibrin, together with moderate numbers of granulocytes. Histologically the picture corresponds to that of a lobar pneumonia in the phase of red hepatization going into gray hepatization (Fig. 18, H & E, 375×).

The history of rupture of the membranes 4 days before delivery, a positive blood culture obtained by catheterization of the umbilical vessels at birth, and the radiologic observations at 4 hours suggest an intrauterine origin of the infection.

As well as by premature rupture of the membranes, as in this case, ascending infection may be caused by prolonged labor or by obstetrical maneuvers. Furthermore, microorganisms can reach the lung of the fetus by the transplacental route.

It is possible to demonstrate the offending organisms in the lung, but generally they are not very numerous. If the pneumonia is produced by staphylococci, the lesions are of the necrotic type in many instances, a fact that is not observed in the presence of other microorganisms.

19
MINIMAL GRANULOCYTIC EXUDATE

Nine hundred and thirty gram male of unknown gestational age. Apgar score 3 at birth. Resuscitation by means of aspiration and administration of oxygen.

Admitted at 1 hour of age, obviously immature, with generalized loss of muscle tone, gasping respiration, cyanosis, and genital edema. Six hours after admission, while receiving 10 per cent glucose intravenously: pH 7.33, pCO_2 68 mm Hg, BE -2 mEq/L. The chest x-ray did not suggest hyaline membrane disease.

The picture of respiratory failure persisted, and death occurred at 20 hours of life during an apneic episode.

Histopathologic Examination. The lung is well expanded, with alveolar spaces of varying sizes and some remaining cuboidal alveolar lining cells. The majority of the capillaries are exposed to the lumen. In this illustration there are clusters of granulocytes occupying parts of the lumina of some alveoli; other alveoli are free of exudate (H & E, 375×).

This picture contrasts markedly with that of intrauterine pneumonia, in which there is more abundant and widespread inflammatory cell infiltration (Figs. 13 and 14), and with that of acquired pneumonia, in which the inflammatory components are different.

Minimal granulocytic exudate is frequently observed in the lungs of premature infants who have suffered serious neonatal anoxia. It is possible that this pattern may correspond to minor forms of intrauterine pneumonia.

In this case there were also extensive subarachnoid hemorrhage and other signs of immaturity, particularly in the kidney and the brain.

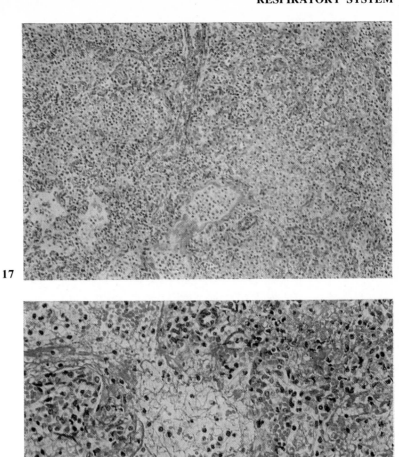

17

18

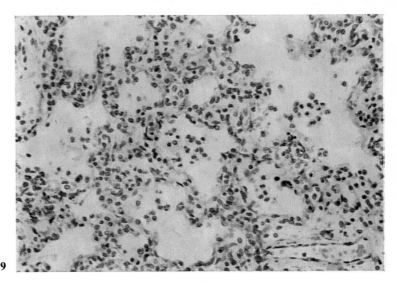

19

20
CONGESTIVE PULMONARY ATELECTASIS

Full-term newborn weighing 3,340 gm at birth. Apgar score 5. Admitted at 4 hours of age with severe respiratory distress and a fracture of the right femur. pH 7.16, pCO_2 91 mm Hg, BE −8.5 mEq/L.

X-ray of the chest showed large unexpanded areas not suggestive of pulmonary hyaline membrane disease. A crisis of apnea at 36 hours forced intubation and the use of assisted ventilation. The pH improved with intravenous administration of bicarbonate. pH 7.36, pCO_2 55 mm Hg, BE +3 mEq/L.

The infant died at 3 days of age in progressive respiratory failure.

Histopathologic Examination. The alveolar spaces are small, and the interalveolar septa are relatively thick, with engorged capillaries. There is no alveolar edema, nor are there any hyaline membranes (H & E, 375×).

Autopsy revealed severe subarachnoid hemorrhage.

21
ACUTE PULMONARY EDEMA ASSOCIATED WITH CONGESTION AND ATELECTASIS

Fifteen hundred gram female with gestational age of 29 weeks. Twenty-two hours of labor. Rupture of membranes 24 hours before delivery. Cephalic presentation. Neonatal anoxia. Resuscitation by means of aspiration and oxygen therapy.

Admitted at 2 hours of life with generalized cyanosis, loss of muscle tone, and muffled cardiac sounds. The infant was placed in an incubator. Oxygen was administered. Acidosis was corrected, but the child died 3 hours after admission.

Histopathologic Examination. The pulmonary parenchyma is atelectatic. There is capillary engorgment. The alveolar ducts are dilated and filled with homogeneous eosinophilic material that stains pink; in some areas the ducts are lined by thin pseudomembranous pink-staining condensations (H & E, 375×).

Grossly, the lungs were wine-red and did not float. There were numerous petechiae over the pleural surfaces, epicardium, kidney, thymus, and meninges.

22
ATELECTASIS AND PULMONARY EDEMA WITH HYALINE MEMBRANES

Male weighing 3,750 gm. Gestational age, 43 weeks. Vertex delivery of 8 hours' duration. Apgar score 8 at birth.

Admitted after 30 minutes with slight respiratory difficulty, which became greater in the succeeding hours, with intense cyanosis that did not yield to the administration of oxygen. At 12 hours an air bronchogram compatible with the diagnosis of pulmonary hyaline membrane disease was observed.

Death occurred 2 hours later.

Histopathologic Examination. The picture is of a relatively early phase of pulmonary atelectasis with hyaline membranes. The alveolar ducts in the center of Figure 22 are very dilated, and the walls are lined by a homogeneous layer of hyaline material that is thin and interrupted and that stands out from the surrounding pulmonary edema because of its greater density and eosinophilic character (H & E, 187.5×).

23
PULMONARY ATELECTASIS WITH HYALINE MEMBRANES

Male weighing 1,960 gm. Gestational age, 36 weeks. Normal delivery, vertex presentation, spontaneous cry.

Admitted at 3 hours with respiratory difficulty and moaning. Chest x-rays showed an air bronchogram and opaque lung fields. Acid-base balance on admission showed: pH 7.12, pCO_2 55.5 mm Hg, BE −7.5 mEq/L.

The patient was treated with an infusion of 10 per cent dextrose and 1 M bicarbonate intravenously, placed in an incubator, and given oxygen.

The picture of respiratory insufficiency continued to worsen. At 48 hours: pH 7.19, pCO_2 77 mm Hg, BE −4 mEq/L.

Death occurred at 60 hours of age in an apneic crisis.

Histopathologic Examination. There are hyaline membranes that completely line the terminal bronchioles and the alveolar ducts. The pulmonary parenchyma shows considerable atelectasis with capillary engorgement. The pattern corresponds to a more advanced stage than that illustrated in the preceding case (H & E, 375×).

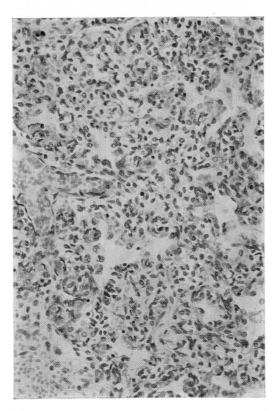

20

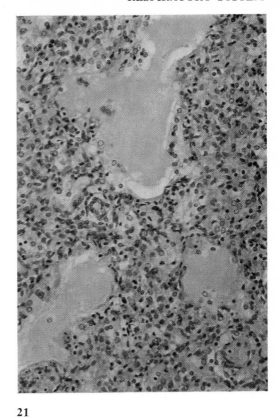

21

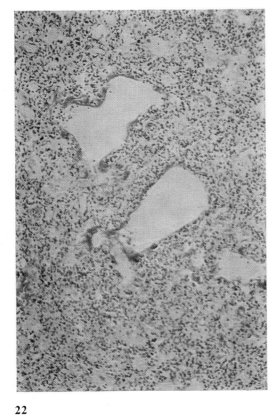

22

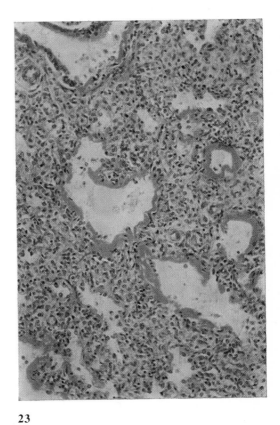

23

HYALINE MEMBRANES WITH NUCLEAR REMNANTS

Seven hundred and fifty gram female. Gestational age, 25 weeks. Twin birth. Breech presentation. Apgar score 1 at 1 minute. Energetic resuscitation.

Admitted at 30 minutes of life in poor general condition with decreased muscle tone and loss of reflexes. Mixed acidosis, respiratory and metabolic. Death occurred 6 hours later as a result of respiratory distress.

Histopathologic Examination. In some places hyaline membranes are amphophilic and contain abundant nuclear remnants, attributable to destroyed alveolar or bronchiolar lining cells. Here abundant hematoxylin-staining spherical bodies may also be found (Fig. 24, H & E, 600×).

Some bronchiolar ducts are also filled with hyaline masses containing abundant nuclear remnants similar to those lining many air spaces. The picture resembles that of obstructive bronchiolitis; it should be pointed out that in this case there is no inflammatory infiltrate either in the walls of bronchioles or in the nearby air spaces; atelectasis is moderate (Fig. 25, H & E, 187.5×).

Illustration 25 pertains to the case of an infant weighing 1,250 gm, 32 weeks' gestation. Born in transverse presentation with manual extraction. Apgar 4. Metabolic acidosis. pH 7.10, pCO_2 27.5 mm Hg, BE −20.5 mEq/L. Death occurred 4 hours after admission.

In our experience, hyaline membranes with nuclear remnants are observed chiefly in very small infants or in those with a history of prolonged or complicated labor and delivery. The interrupted character of the membranes and their varying thickness should be emphasized.

ATELECTASIS WITH HYALINE MEMBRANES

Male weighing 1,900 gm. First born of a twin delivery. Gestational age, 28 weeks. Breech presentation. Five hour delivery. Single placenta. Apgar score 9 at birth. Required no resuscitation, but merely aspiration of mucous secretions.

On admission at 5 hours of life, he showed generalized cyanosis and respiratory wheeze.

The x-ray of the chest showed a typical air bronchogram, and the diagnosis of pulmonary hyaline membrane disease was established. pH 7.18, pCO_2 56 mm Hg, BE −9 mEq/L.

Treatment with 10 per cent dextrose and 1 M bicarbonate was instituted for correction of the acidosis. Cyanosis did not yield to the administration of 100 per cent oxygen. The picture of respiratory insufficiency became progressive, and the infant died at 48 hours of age.

Histopathologic Examination. Conventional microscopic examination showed this to be a case of typical pulmonary hyaline membranes with atelectasis.

Fluorescence studies with acridine orange show intense green fluorescence of the hyaline membranes. The air spaces appear black, and the remainder of the parenchyma exhibits golden fluorescence of the nuclei (Fig. 26, 600×).

Incubation of sections of fresh lung prepared with the cryostat and labeled with antifibrinogen–fluoresceine isothiocyanate demonstrates specific fluorescence of the hyaline membranes, identifying fibrinogen as an important component of the latter (Fig. 27, 600×). With alpha-1-anti-trypsin labeled antiserum, the presence of an important deposit of this substance within the hyaline membranes is also demonstrated with a fluorescence intensity comparable to that noted with antifibrinogen.

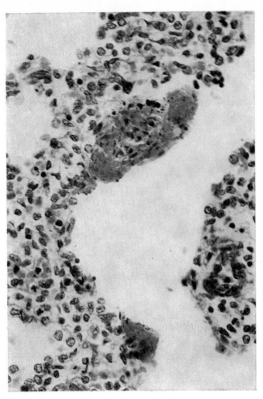

24

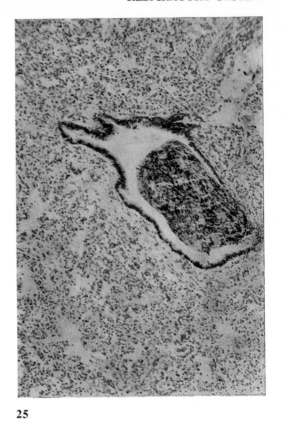

25

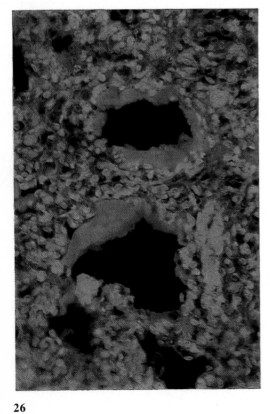

26

27

PULMONARY HYALINE MEMBRANES IN PROCESS OF RESORPTION

Fifteen hundred and fifty gram male. 38 week gestation. Breech presentation. Apgar score 9 at birth.

Admitted at 2 hours of age in good general condition. Eight hours after admission respiratory insufficiency began. pH 7.05, pCO 73 mm Hg, BE −11.5 mEq/L.

An intravenous infusion of 10 per cent dextrose and 1 M bicarbonate was started. Chest x-rays showed the typical signs of pulmonary hyaline membrane disease in the form of an air bronchogram. Respiratory insufficiency progressed. At 72 hours: pH 7.14, pCO_2 80 mm Hg, BE +6 mEq/L. Crises of apnea recurred, and death ensued on the fifth day of life.

Histopathologic Examination. The illustration shows marked atelectasis with dilated capillaries. The thick hyaline membranes that line the air spaces are partially fragmented (Fig. 28, H & E, 600×).

There are macrophages in the air spaces. Epithelization over the surface of the membranes, which are partly fused with the alveolar walls, is noteworthy. (Fig. 29, H & E, 375×).

The absence of polymorphonuclear leukocytes as an inflammatory element in any of the sections is striking, inasmuch as the infant died at the age of five days.

30
RESIDUAL PULMONARY LESIONS FOLLOWING A CLINICAL PICTURE OF HYALINE MEMBRANE DISEASE

Female, weighing 2,000 gm. Gestational age, 36 weeks. Apgar score 7. The infant was admitted at 6 hours of life with respiratory difficulty. The radiographic pattern at 12 hours was typical of pulmonary hyaline membranes. pH 7.21, pCO_2 73 mm Hg, BE −3 mEq/L.

The pO_2 values in an atmosphere of 50 per cent oxygen were 45 mm Hg, and in 100 per cent oxygen, 80 mm Hg. Periods of apnea forced the use of intubation and assisted respiration. Assisted respiration had to be maintained for 6 days. The pO_2 values in 100 per cent oxygen atmosphere hovered between 65 and 75 mm Hg.

Death occurred 6 days postnatally.

Histopathologic Examination. The interalveolar septa are thickened and edematous, with early signs of fibrosis. There is also moderate swelling of the lining epithelial cells. There are numerous erythrocytes in the alveolar lumina (Masson, 375×).

There were no important findings in other organs except for moderate cerebral congestion and edema.

Pulmonary lesions of this type are probably attributable to oxygen therapy and represent so-called bronchopulmonary dysplasia (see Figs. 101 and 102).

31
BRONCHOPNEUMONIA IN A NEWBORN WITH PULMONARY HYALINE MEMBRANES

A 2,300 gm female. Gestational age, 36 weeks. Admitted at 8 hours of age. Rupture of membranes 2 days before delivery. Vertex presentation.

On admission, physical examination was apparently normal. At 15 hours of age respiratory distress began, with subcostal retraction, tachypnea, and cyanosis. Studies of acid-base balance showed pH 7.10, pCO_2 55 mm Hg, BE −10 mEq/L. Chest x-ray showed the presence of an air bronchogram and a diffuse reticulonodular picture in the lung fields bilaterally. Treatment in an incubator with oxygen therapy and an infusion of 10 per cent glucose with bicarbonate was ineffectual. Respiratory failure worsened; pH 7.18, pCO_2 69 mm Hg, BE −3 mEq/L.

Death occurred at 54 hours.

Histopathologic Examination. Together with typical hyaline membranes there are residual areas of atelectasis. The majority of the air spaces in Figure 31 are dilated and contain dense accumulations of polymorphonuclear leukocytes (H & E, 375×).

The presence of isolated polymorphonuclear leukocytes without any infectious component is frequently observed in infants who die between 36 and 48 hours after the onset of respiratory distress associated with pulmonary hyaline membranes. It is, however, unlikely that the inflammatory cells are related to resorption of the hyaline membranes; rather, they are the result of a superimposed infection. The density of the inflammatory infiltrate in the present case leads to the assumption that this represents bronchopneumonia.

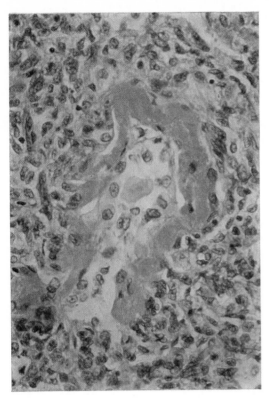

28

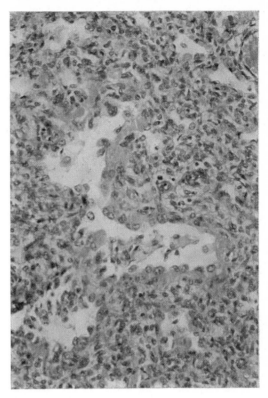

29

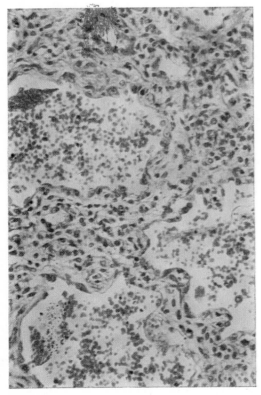

30

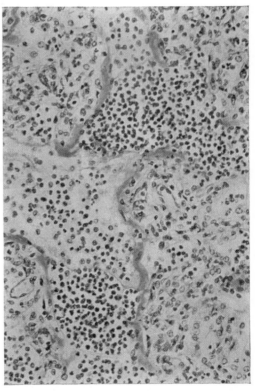

31

PERIVASCULAR HEMORRHAGE DUE TO DIAPEDESIS

A 2,400 gm male. Unknown gestational age. Delivery took place in a taxi as the mother was being brought to a hospital.

On admission, at 2 hours of life, the infant was in poor general condition with cyanosis, hypotonia, gasping respirations, and inadequate response to stimuli.

Death occurred in a few minutes in spite of resuscitative efforts.

Histopathologic Examination. In addition to congestion and atelectasis involving both lungs, perivascular hemorrhages resulting from diapedesis probably attributable to anoxia can be observed. Note the absence of blood in air spaces (H & E, 187.5×).

Other findings in the autopsy included bilateral hydronephrosis with megaloureter and posterior urethral valves.

33/34

INTRAALVEOLAR PULMONARY HEMORRHAGE

Female weighing 1,500 gm. Unknown gestational age. Mother hypertensive during pregnancy. Vertex presentation. Apgar score 5 at birth.

Admitted 1 hour postnatally. Examination showed facial edema, hypotonia, and serosanguineous collections in the subcutaneous tissues of the occipital and frontoparietal areas. Ten per cent glucose solution was given intravenously, and the infant was placed in an incubator. Within 24 hours there had been notable improvement. At 48 hours, however, an episode of apnea occurred. Acid-base balance showed, at that time, the presence of mixed acidosis with pH 7.12, pCO_2 57 mm Hg, BE −16 mEq/L.

1 M bicarbonate was added to the intravenous infusion. Two hours later apnea recurred with intense cyanosis and hematemesis. In spite of resuscitative measures death took place at 56 hours.

Histopathologic Examination. Marked alveolar collapse with thickening of septa and mas-

sive filling of air spaces in all the lobes by blood was observed. The hemorrhage was selectively intraalveolar and intrabronchiolar; there was no concomitant inflammatory component. Note the dilatation of lymphatics in the perilobular septa (Fig. 33, H & E, 60×).

There was also subarachnoid hemorrhage limited to the right parietooccipital region.

Figure 34 shows intraalveolar hemorrhage of massive proportions in a 1,660 gram male (H & E, 187.5×). Gestational age, 29 weeks. The clinical course was satisfactory until the fifth day of life, when suddenly, respiratory insufficiency with apnea, cyanosis, and the expulsion of blood and serosanguineous mucus from the mouth and nose occurred, accompanied by mixed acidosis with pH 6.72, pCO_2 12 mm Hg, and BE −21 mEq/L. The infant died 2 hours later.

The term "hemorrhagic pneumonia of the newborn" is not really accurate when applied to lesions such as this, inasmuch as the cause of the hemorrhage is not inflammatory. On the other hand, the alveolar septa are well preserved and clearly visible (Fig. 34), and the architecture of the lung is normal, contrary to what might be expected were infarction present.

35

SUBPLEURAL AND SEPTAL HEMORRHAGE

Male weighing 2,000 gm. Unknown gestational age. Admitted at 6 hours of life in terminal condition with gasping respiration, hypothermia, bradycardia, atony, and pallor. Death occurred at the moment of admission.

Histopathologic Examination. Figure 35 shows hemorrhagic infiltration of the pleura, which is thickened at this level. This hemorrhage continues into the interlobular connective tissue. There are no intraalveolar hemorrhagic foci (H & E, 17.5×). In other fields there were polymorphonuclear leukocytes in the alveolar lumina with the characteristics of an intrauterine pneumonia.

Autopsy further disclosed massive subarachnoid hemorrhage as well as multiple scattered petechiae.

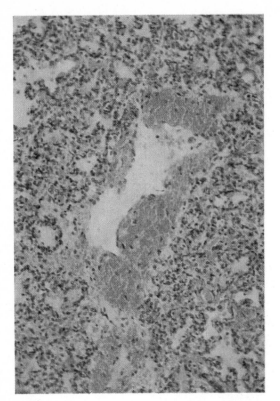

32

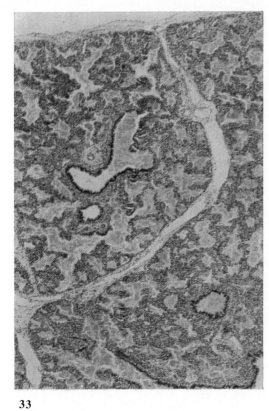

33

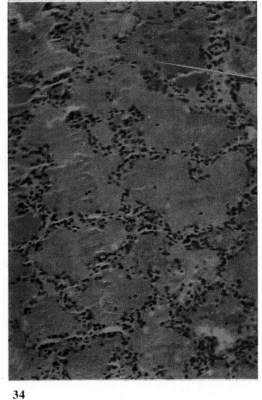

34

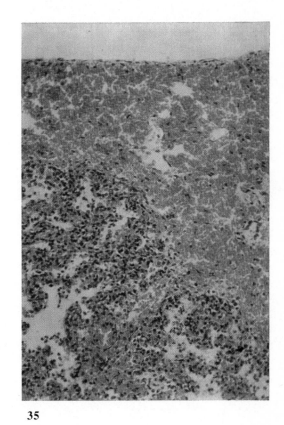

35

MASSIVE PULMONARY HEMORRHAGE

A 2,900 gm male. Unknown gestational age, twin birth. Forceps delivery. Apgar score 9 at birth. Expiratory whine on admission at 3 hours of age. Mild cyanosis disappeared with the administration of oxygen. Ten per cent glucose solution was given.

Normal acid-base balance. Favorable course until 48 hours of age, at which time blood was ejected through nose and mouth, and apnea and cyanosis appeared. In spite of resuscitation including aspiration, the infant died.

Histopathologic Examination. Figure 36 shows a septal vessel with dilated lumen; its branches are also dilated and communicate with an area of intraalveolar hemorrhage that occupies the greater part of a lobule (Masson, 60×).

In another field the alveolar pattern has disappeared completely in the hemorrhagic areas (Fig. 37, Masson, 187.5×).

Other sections showed associated lesions, including aspiration of amniotic fluid and meconium with a mild granulocytic reaction.

The frequency of pulmonary hemorrhage as a cause of death in a recent series of 700 autopsies on newborns in the first 30 days of life was 10.6 per cent for full-term infants and 17.9 per cent for prematures.

DISSECTING ANEURYSM OF A PULMONARY VESSEL

Male weighing 3,200 gm. Gestational age, 40 weeks. Apgar score 10. Clinical diagnosis was esophageal atresia with distal tracheoesophageal fistula and imperforate anus with fistula. Convulsions occurred at 24 hours of age. Spinal fluid bacteriologically negative. Palpable mass in right side of abdomen.

Intravenous urogram showed a single renal shadow with paired calices, pelves, and ureters. Blood urea, 155 mg/100 ml. Death intervened at 48 hours of age.

Histopathologic Examination. Figure 38 shows a dissecting aneurysm of a pulmonary vessel. The diameter of the vessel is increased as a result of a collection of blood that has dissected the adventitia away from the muscular coat. The lumen is collapsed and occluded (H & E, 187.5×).

The child showed bacterial bronchopneumonia associated with esophageal atresia and tracheoesophageal fistula. In addition, the left kidney was located on the right side and fused with the other kidney, each having its own excretory system. There was also an imperforate anus with a rectoperineal fistula.

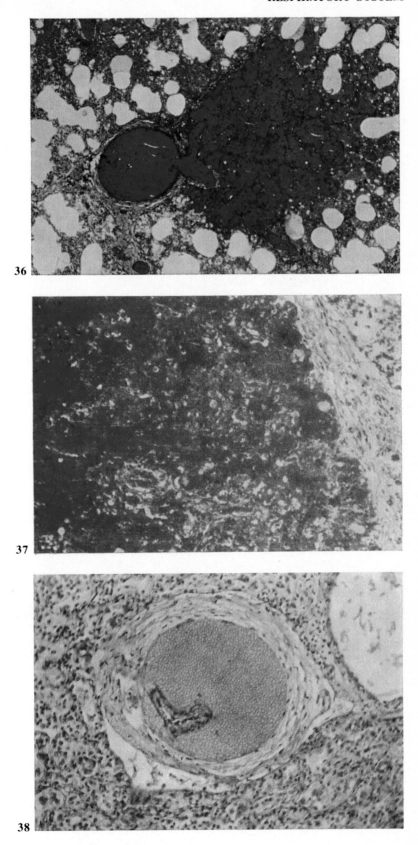

39
PSEUDOPOLYPOID TRACHEITIS

Two thousand seven hundred gram male; gestational age, 38 weeks. Vertex delivery after 6 hours of labor. Severe anoxia at birth requiring resuscitation with aspiration, intubation, and oxygen therapy.

Admitted 3 hours later in poor general condition, pale, and with decreased muscle tone. He was put in an incubator and given 10 per cent dextrose and antibiotics intravenously. Metabolic acidosis with pH 7.13, pCO_2 27 mm Hg, BE −9 mEq/L. Bicarbonate infusion corrected that situation. Respiratory distress increased in the succeeding hours, and chest x-ray showed poor aeration of the right apex and coarse hilar markings. Culture of gastric contents was negative.

Treatment with antibiotics, dextrose, and bicarbonate was continued by umbilical catheter. pH 7.10, pCO_2 71 mm Hg, BE −10.5 mEq/L.

The course was downhill, with apneic bouts and generalized cyanosis leading to the necessity for controlled assisted respiration. Death occurred at 60 hours of life.

Histopathologic Examination. Figure 39 represents a section of trachea. There is a polypoid structure with loss of surface epithelium projecting into the lumen. The body of the "polyp" consists of granulation tissue with hyaline thrombi filling the capillaries and infiltration by round cells and polymorphonuclear leukocytes (H & E, 600×). The lesion is probably iatrogenic and attributable to intubation. There was also extensive subarachnoid hemorrhage.

40
ACUTE FIBRINOPURULENT BRONCHIOLITIS

Twenty-two day old male weighing 2,000 gm. Admitted for diarrhea and respiratory difficulty with coughing of 3 days' duration. On admission, he was in serious general condition, with respiratory distress, tachypnea, moaning, and dehydration. pH 7.18, pCO_2 50.5 mm Hg, BE −9.2 mEq/L, sodium 176 mEq/L, chloride 154 mEq/L, potassium 6.4 mEq/L, hematocrit 40 per cent. Negative chest x-ray.

In spite of antibiotics and attempts to correct the acidosis, he died in 48 hours. Terminal values were: pH 7.16, pCO_2 62 mm Hg, BE −8.5 mEq/L, chloride 108 mEq/L, sodium 144 mEq/L, potassium 4.5 mEq/L.

Histopathologic Examination. Figure 40 shows the lumen of a terminal or preterminal bronchiole that is occluded by fibrinous masses mingled with polynuclear leukocytes that tend to accumulate along the walls of the alveolar duct and protrude into adjacent alveoli. The lining epithelium is largely destroyed. (H & E, 375×). A similar picture was seen in all lobes.

41
BRONCHIOLITIS OBLITERANS

Female weighing 1,950 gm at birth. Gestational age, 36 weeks. Early development was normal, and she was discharged at 1 month of age with a weight of 2,550 gm. Ten days later she was readmitted with gastroenteritis, isotonic dehydration, metabolic acidosis, respiratory insufficiency, and generalized sepsis.

Stool culture, using differential media, showed colonies of *Candida albicans* and type 0:111/B:4 enteropathogenic *E. coli.* Blood culture was positive for *E. coli,* 1 colony per milliliter of planted blood. The septic manifestations worsened; severe signs of respiratory failure appeared, and the infant died on the sixth hospital day.

Histopathologic Examination. At the center, Figure 41 shows a bronchiole. The lumen, lined by cylindrical epithelium, contains mucus with a moderate number of inflammatory cells. The obstructing material is not adherent to the intact lining epithelium. There is moderate infiltration of the bronchiolar wall by round cells, and nearby desquamative alveolitis (H & E, 187.5×).

Autopsy showed ulcerative, necrotizing enteritis with reactive hepatitis and moderate cholestasis.

Bronchiolitis in the neonatal period is of dubious significance. It is debatable whether it represents an infection (bacterial or viral) or whether it is related to assisted respiration or oxygen therapy or both.

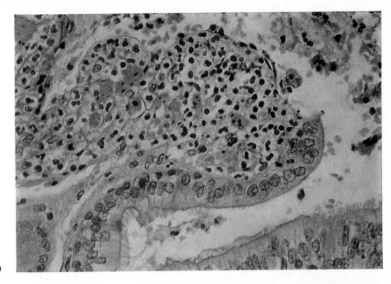

39

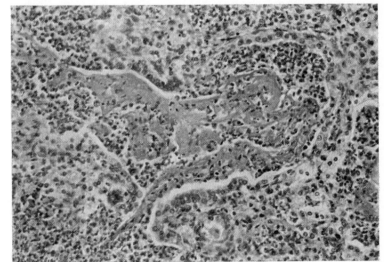

40

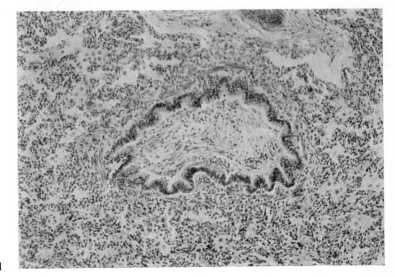

41

GIANT CELL BRONCHIOLITIS

Female weighing 2,000 gm. Gestational age, 34 weeks. Esophageal atresia and low tracheoesophageal fistula, admitted on the fourth day of life in poor general condition with mild signs of respiratory difficulty. Radiography confirmed the presence of esophageal atresia and showed evidence of exudative and atelectatic changes in both lung fields.

After treatment with antibiotics and management of acid-base imbalance, surgery was undertaken on the fifth day of life. Two hours after the operation the infant required endotracheal intubation with assisted respiration. Twenty-four hours later spontaneous respirations appeared, and the mechanical devices were withdrawn. In the course of the next few days, however, respiratory insufficiency began again and became progressively worse; the child died in an apneic episode at 8 days of age.

Histopathologic Examination. In Figure 42 the lumen of the bronchiole appears plugged with polymorphonuclear leukocytes. The most striking feature is the conspicuous alteration of the bronchiolar epithelium (H & E, 187.5×). Under high magnification the epithelial cells appear to be transformed into giant multinucleated units. Some of them show acidophilic inclusion bodies. In other bronchioles the lumen is largely occupied by desquamated giant cells (Fig. 43, H & E, 1,500×).

There were also areas of hemorrhagic pneumonia with remnants of foreign material and reactive pleuritis. The alveoli showed no giant cells.

NECROTIZING DESQUAMATIVE INTERSTITIAL PNEUMONIA

Twenty day old male weighing 3,200 gm transferred from another hospital where he had been admitted for gastroenteritis accompanied by severe metabolic acidosis and gram-negative sepsis without further bacterial identification. Transfer was prompted by the onset of a hemorrhagic syndrome with hemoptysis and cutaneous hemorrhage.

On admission he was in poor general condition with palpebral edema and swelling of the lower extremities. The liver was enlarged by 3 fingerbreadths, and there was mild respiratory insufficiency: pH 7.17, pCO_2 43 mm Hg, BE -12 mEq/L, hematocrit 47 per cent, chloride 105 mEq/L, sodium 130 mEq/L, potassium 4.5 mEq/L. Cultures of blood, gastric contents, and urine were negative. Cerebrospinal fluid culture negative. Feces: Positive culture for enteropathogenic type 0:55/B:5 *E. coli,* positive benzidine test. Coagulation studies normal. Platelets 102,000. Transaminases: SGOT 220 u/L, SGPT 250 u/L.

In spite of treatment for acidosis and gastroenteritis, respiratory insufficiency progressed. Chest x-rays showed generalized emphysema and uniformly scattered fine nodularity in both lung fields.

Respiratory difficulties increased in the following days, and acid-base studies were reported as: pH 7.3, pCO_2 53 mm Hg, BE -2 mEq/L. Nineteen days after admission his general condition appeared worse. There were bouts of apnea and cyanosis; pCO_2 values climbed, and intubation with assisted respiration was employed.

Chest x-rays showed disseminated foci of consolidation over both lung fields and a rounded area of hyperlucency in the periphery of the right lung field. pH 7.25, pCO_2 78 mm Hg, BE $+2$ mEq/L. Death occurred 2 days later.

Histopathologic Examination. Three characteristics stood out in microscopic study of the lung: (1) infiltration of the alveolar septa by round cells, predominantly lymphocytic (Fig. 44, H & E, 187.5×); (2) prominent swelling of the alveolar epithelium as seen in the upper part of Figure 45 (H & E, 600×); and (3) alveolar spaces filled with mostly necrotic PAS positive mononuclear cells with clumped cytoplasm.

In these areas, representing the greater part of the lung, no organisms were demonstrated and methenamine silver stain was negative. There were no inclusion bodies.

There was also bronchopneumonia with a tendency to abscess formation. Other findings included hemorrhagic enteritis and *Candida* esophagitis.

This atypical form of interstitial pneumonitis differs from Liebow's desquamative interstitial pneumonitis by virtue of the necrosis of desquamated alveolar cells, which appear for the most part as "shadows," and the considerable interstitial component. The hilar lymph nodes showed hyperplasia of the thymic-dependent paracortical zone featuring many "blast" forms (large activated lymphocytes).

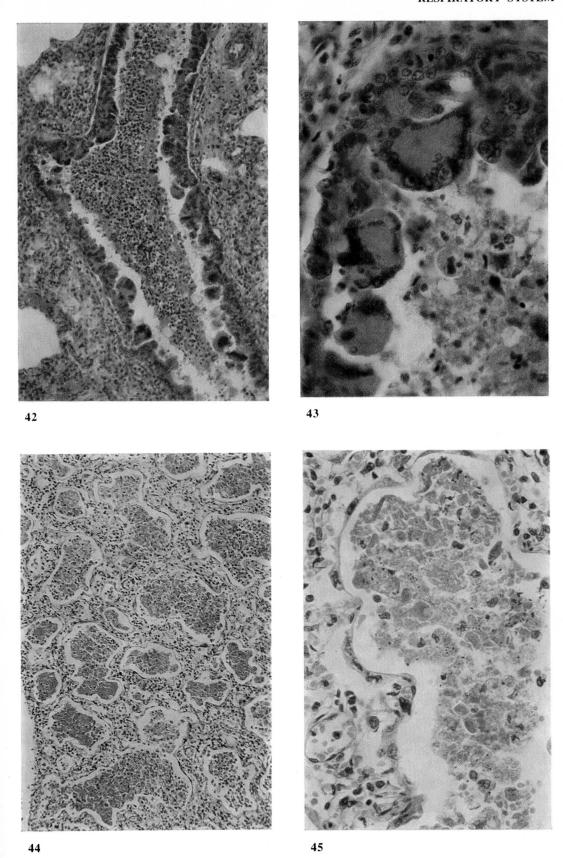

42

43

44

45

ACUTE EPIGLOTTITIS

Twenty-six day old male weighing 3,000 gm at birth. Low-grade fever, rhinitis, and adenoiditis of 1 week's duration. This was followed by respiratory insufficiency and expiratory whine. The former became increasingly worse, and the child was admitted in moribund condition. At that time there was vascular collapse with hyperthermia, dehydration, and respiratory failure. Death occurred immediately.

Histopathologic Examination. Grossly, the larynx, and particularly the epiglottis, showed reddening, tumefaction, and edema, with consequent narrowing of the lumen. Microscopically, the mucosa of the epiglottis shows partial loss of the surface epithelium. The lamina propria is greatly thickened with granulocytic infiltration and areas of fibrinoid necrosis, both near the surface and in deeper zones. Some of the capillaries are thrombosed (Fig. 46, H & E, 187.5×). There were no inflammatory changes in the remainder of the upper respiratory tract nor in the obviously emphysematous lungs. Figure 47 shows a simple acute epiglottitis with more subdued changes, preservation of the surface epithelium, and edema with inflammatory infiltration in the lamina propria (H & E, 187.5×). This illustration corresponds to a 15 day old infant who presented with acute respiratory distress following the aspiration of a nipple and succumbed upon admission to the hospital. Autopsy revealed acute epiglottitis, focal interstitial granulocytic pneumonitis, acute pulmonary edema, and terminal aspiration of milk.

PERIPHERAL PULMONARY ATELECTASIS

Female weighing 1,140 gm. Unknown gestational age. Normal vertex delivery. Apgar 6 at 1 minute after birth.

Admitted 3 hours later with moderate cyanosis, slight distal edema, and hypotonia.

Chest x-ray at 24 hours showed no evidence of hyaline membrane disease but rather marked hyperlucency of both lung fields. pH 7.24, pCO_2 45 mm Hg, BE −8.5 mEq/L.

After treatment the infant's condition improved for 48 hours, but later respiratory insufficiency and acidosis recurred. pH 7.24, pCO_2 54 mm Hg, BE −6 mEq/L. Jaundice appeared. Total bilirubin 19.7 mg/100 ml with no evidence of isoimmunization. Death intervened 4 hours later.

Histopathologic Examination. Figure 48 shows marked dilatation of most alveolar ducts and a terminal bronchiole (lower left), contrasting with the atelectasis of adjacent parenchyma. There are also groups of tubular spaces. The septal capillaries are markedly dilated (H & E, 60×). This type of overinsufflation is seen with some frequency following energetic resuscitative maneuvers involving immature lungs. Gruenwald considers this to represent "exaggerated atelectasis of prematurity" in the recuperative phase of respiratory distress syndrome in prematures.

Figure 49 shows pulmonary atelectasis with marked dilatation limited to the terminal portions of the respiratory bronchioles and the alveolar ducts, contrasting with collapse of remaining parenchyma (H & E, 187.5×).

The patient was a 950 gm infant of 28 weeks' gestation with an Apgar score of 5 at birth. An apneic crisis dictated resuscitation. Generalized cyanosis and hypotony ensued, followed by death at 3 hours (see also Figs. 15 and 16).

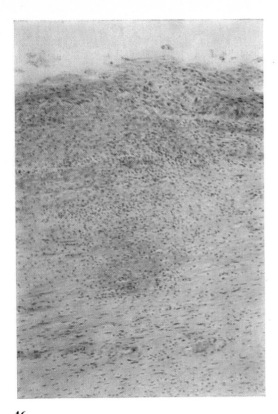

46

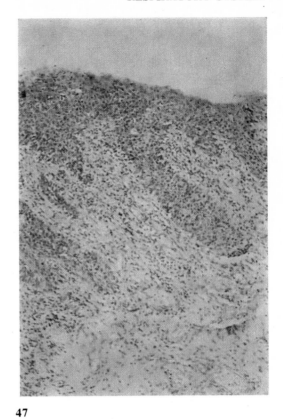

47

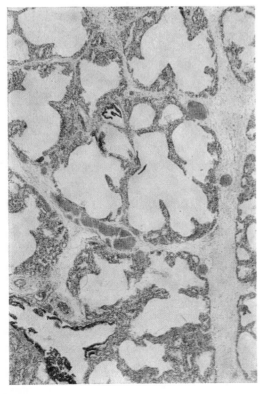

48

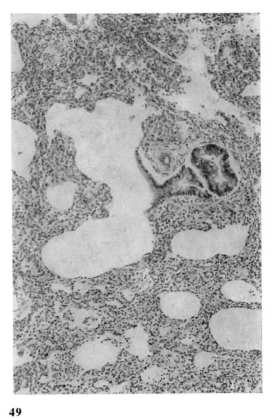

49

PULMONARY ABSCESSES FOLLOWING ASPIRATION

Male weighing 2,360 gm. Gestational age, 36 weeks. Admitted at 10 hours of life. Precipitous vertex delivery. No spontaneous cry on delivery. Mucus was aspirated and oxygen therapy administered.

At 7 hours there was accumulation of secretions in the oral cavity with generalized cyanosis, expiratory whine, depressed reflexes, and irregular breathing. Death ensued 5 hours after admission from progressive respiratory failure with cyanosis and refractory apnea.

Histopathologic Examination. Figure 50 shows a subpleural, roughly wedge-shaped necrotizing inflammatory focus adjacent to bronchial branches. In the midst of the lesion, destruction of alveolar septa is evident accompanied by granulocytic infiltration and bacterial colonies. The lumen of the bronchiole is plugged by leukocytes (H & E, 60×). Similar foci were scattered over the greater part of the surface of the lung.

Considering the short term of life of the infant (12 hours), the advanced stage of the lesions is striking. It is possible that these rapidly evolving necrotizing lesions might be related to aspiration of maternal feces.

Autopsy also revealed extensive subarachnoid hemorrhage over the cerebellar hemispheres. There were no signs of generalized sepsis.

ASPIRATION AND ACUTE EMPHYSEMA

Female weighing 4,200 gm. Gestational age, 42 weeks. Three hour labor, vertex delivery.

Physical examination revealed anencephaly, respiratory distress and intense cyanosis, expiratory whine, and weak response to stimuli. Death at 40 hours.

Histopathologic Examination. Brownish material had been aspirated and was associated with marked pulmonary emphysema. Alveolar septa were ruptured, and large air-filled cavities had formed (Figs. 51 and 52, H & E, 375×).

There was also bilateral renal and adrenal hypoplasia. The weight of the lungs was normal.

Aspiration of foreign matter, especially of alimentary origin, gives rise to four basic types of change. Sometimes, as in the present case, it causes acute pulmonary hyperinsufflation because of bronchial obstruction. It can also lead to bronchopneumonia (Figs. 53 and 54), frequently with abscess formation (inhalation abscesses). Less commonly the foreign material will provoke the formation of micronodular granulomatous lesions featuring foreign body giant cells (Figs. 55 and 56). Finally, if the aspirated material contains fatty substances (milk, fat-soluble vitamins) the picture of lipoid pneumonia may be produced (Figs. 59 and 60).

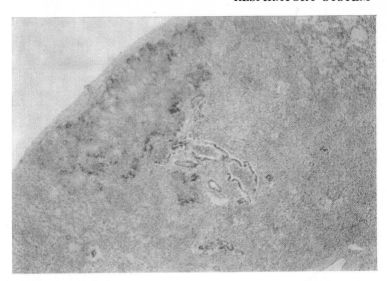

50

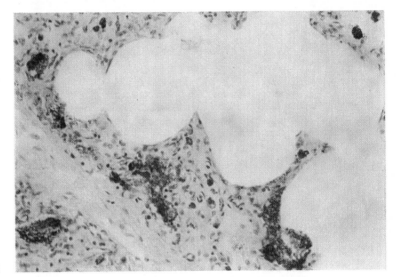

51

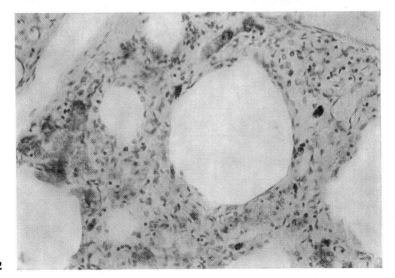

52

53/54
PNEUMONIA ASSOCIATED WITH ASPIRATION OF FOOD

Female weighing 2,300 gm. Gestational age, 39 weeks. Labor of 3 hours' duration followed by vertex delivery. Apgar score 9 at birth. Admitted at 48 hours in poor general condition with generalized cyanosis and epidermolysis bullosa. Culture of the fluid in the bullae was negative.

At four days of life signs of respiratory failure appeared, manifested by an expiratory whine. X-rays showed confluent nodular densities compatible with the diagnosis of bronchopneumonia.

Respiratory failure persisted. After several bouts of cyanosis and apnea the infant died at 20 days of life.

Histopathologic Examination. Figure 53 shows alveolar spaces filled with polynuclear leukocytes mingled with particles of a foreign substance (H & E, 375×).

The bronchioles, shown in Figure 54, are dilated and contain amorphous material as well as vegetable cells; there is no inflammatory reaction, which suggests a terminal bout of inhalation (H & E, 375×).

This may represent aspiration of a vegetable such as carrots or a vegetable preparation employed as an additive in formula.

55/56
PULMONARY GRANULOMATOSIS INDUCED BY VEGETABLE MATTER

Male weighing 2,400 gm. Gestational age, 35 weeks. Birth by breech presentation. Four hour labor. Apgar score 6 at birth.

Admitted at 4 hours of life in poor general condition, with hypotonia and cyanosis. Ulcerated myelomeningocele, hare lip, and cleft palate were noted. Four hours later the myelomeningocele was corrected surgically with ablation of the neural plate.

The postoperative course was stormy, punctuated by respiratory problems, which subsided a few days later.

Two weeks after the operation diarrhea developed, followed by dehydration and metabolic acidosis (pH 7.14, pCO_2 34 mm Hg, BE −20.8 mEq/L), necessitating controlled rehydration. Culture of feces was negative.

Two days later the respiratory difficulties recurred, then worsened. Chest x-rays showed small, confluent nodular densities. Death occurred at 29 days of age.

Histopathologic Examination. Microscopic examination of the lung demonstrates foci of bronchopneumonia with polynuclear infiltration. In Figure 55 the presence of vegetable remnants deeply stained by the PAS method is obvious. They are surrounded by macrophages (600×).

Figure 56 corresponds to a nodular lesion with vegetable cells in the center surrounded by foreign body giant cells. More peripherally there are fibroblasts that tend to form a sort of capsule (H & E, 375×).

In this case the source of the vegetable cells was thought to be diluted carrot juice that had been used as an expander in the milk formula. Pulmonary granulomas have also been described in connection with grain and bean products.

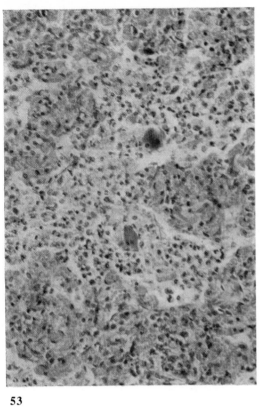

53

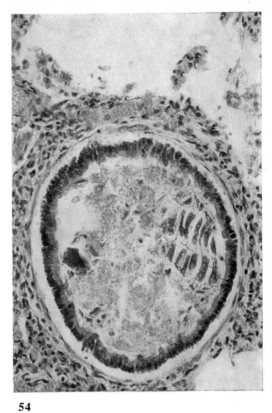

54

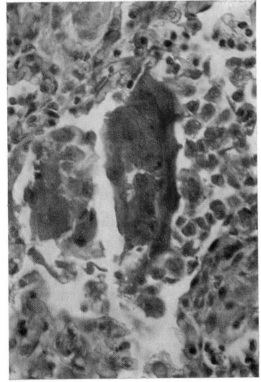

55

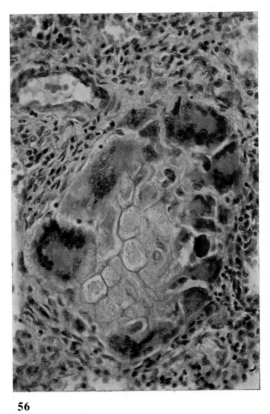

56

57/58
DESQUAMATIVE ALVEOLITIS

Male weighing 2,400 gm. Gestational age, 35 weeks. This is the same case as that presented for Figures 55 and 56.

Histopathologic Examination. In addition to the aspiration pneumonia, there are lumps of desquamated alveolar cells filling air spaces. These cells have light pink-staining cytoplasm. (Stains for fat, iron, and PAS reactive substances were negative.) There is no septal inflammatory infiltration in these areas (Fig. 57, H & E, 375×). In some fields squames can be seen, together with an occasional multinucleated giant cell (Fig. 58, H & E, 375×).

The alveolar lining cells in this case can be interpreted as responding in phagocytic reaction to aspirated material, the aspiration being the result of swallowing difficulties occasioned by the cleft palate.

59/60
LIPOID PNEUMONIA

Twenty-five day old female weighing 3,500 gm, admitted as an emergency with a three day history of dyspnea, cough, and refusal to nurse. These symptoms had become alarmingly more severe within the preceding 24 hours. On examination, signs of severe cardiac decompensation were noted that were attributed to congenital heart disease.

Cardiologic studies pointed to an ample interventricular septal defect. In the next few hours respiratory distress increased. Chest radiographs showed cardiac enlargement and also right-sided pneumothorax. Correction of the latter was attempted by means of closed drainage. Incidentally there was a history of easy regurgitation of food.

Death followed an episode of respiratory arrest 2 days later.

Histopathologic Examination. The alveolar spaces contain many large macrophages with foamy cytoplasm, erythrocytes and some granulocytes. The septal capillaries are dilated and septal cells are prominent (Fig. 59, H & E, 600×).

Sudan III stain demonstrates the lipid character of the phagocytized particles within the alveoli. Some septal macrophages also contain fat (Fig. 60, 600×).

The history of repeated regurgitation argues for the exogenous origin of the lipid material (aspiration of milk).

Autopsy confirmed the presence of an interventricular septal defect 1.4 cm in diameter.

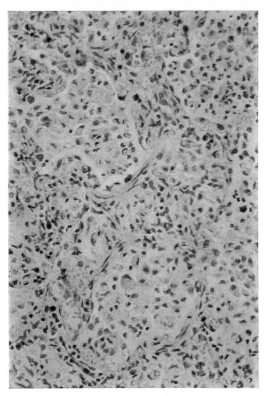

57

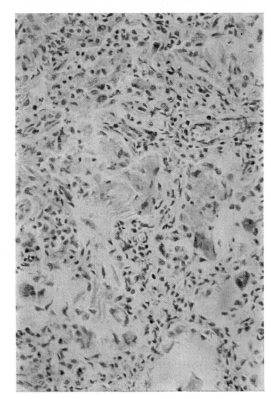

58

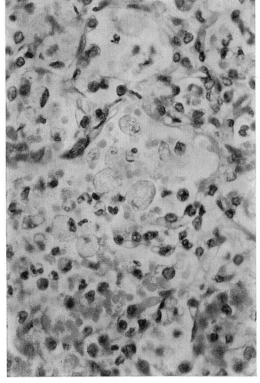

59

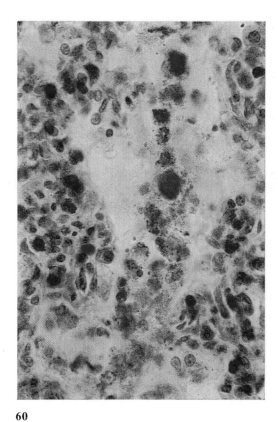

60

61
PSEUDOMONAS PNEUMONIA

Nine day old female weighing 3,200 gm, admitted because of liquid stools and vomiting. She had been receiving hyperconcentrated feedings. Her general condition was poor, with dry oral mucosa, grayish pallor, and acidotic breath. The skin retained a pinch fold. pH 7.20, pCO_2 34 mm Hg, BE −12 mEq/L, plasma chloride 126 mEq/L, sodium 146 mEq/L, potassium 5.8 mEq/L, osmolarity 365 mOsm/L, microhematocrit 43 per cent, total protein 7.6 gm/100 ml.

In spite of treatment for hypertonic dehydration, severe acidosis continued and signs of respiratory failure appeared. X-rays showed nodular confluent bronchopneumonic foci. pH 7.03, pCO_2 54 mm Hg, BE −17 mEq/L. Blood culture was positive for *Pseudomonas,* and fluid taken from a blister on the scalp was positive for the same organism. Clinical course continued to be unfavorable. Necrotic lesions appeared in the left ear; the platelet count decreased and there were anoxic crises; 5 days after admission she died.

Histopathologic Examination. Figure 61 shows a well-defined area of necrosis around a vessel the walls of which are necrotic and contain colonies of organisms that proved to be gram-negative. The lumen of the vessel is obliterated by a thrombus. Note the rather sparse inflammatory reaction (H & E, 187.5×).

Postmortem cultures of pleural fluid, lung, kidney, and liver on blood-agar plates produced innumerable colonies of organisms identifiable as *Pseudomonas aeruginosa.*

62
BACTERIAL PNEUMONIA

Female weighing 1,500 gm. Unknown gestational age. Delivered at home by vertex presentation. Brought to clinic in poor sanitary condition 4 hours after birth.

On admission there was respiratory distress, acrocyanosis, loss of muscle tone, abdominal distention, and poor general condition. Acidosis, with these values: pH 7.16, pCO_2 63 mm Hg, BE −7.5 mEq/L. In the ensuing days respiratory difficulty increased, and a number of arrests necessitated resuscitative measures. Chest x-rays showed scattered and confluent nodular densities, especially in the right lung field.

Death occurred on the fifth hospital day.

Histopathologic Examination. The alveolar spaces and the bronchiolar lumina are occupied by granulocytic exudate. The alveolar septa are thickened and themselves infiltrated by inflammatory cells without being engorged. A moderate number of erythrocytes are mingled with the exudate in some alveoli (H & E, 187.5×).

Grossly, the areas of consolidation represented about 75 per cent of the pulmonary parenchyma. There was also subarachnoid hemorrhage, involving predominantly the posterior portion of the left hemisphere.

63
KLEBSIELLA PNEUMONIAE ARTERITIS

Male weighing 2,600 gm. Gestational age, 37 weeks. Vertex presentation. Apgar score 10 at birth. A nonulcerated myelomeningocele was surgically corrected. Eight days later the diameter of the head was found to have increased, and a pneumoencephalogram confirmed the presence of hydrocephalus; a Holter valve was implanted. The subsequent course was good until the twenty-sixth day, at which time diarrhea and metabolic acidosis occurred with general deterioration and signs of respiratory difficulty. Culture of gastric contents yielded *Klebsiella pneumoniae* and *Proteus.* Blood culture was positive for *Klebsiella,* and urine culture for *Candida, Klebsiella,* and *Proteus.* The infant's condition worsened; respiratory difficulties continued, and hemorrhagic infiltration appeared under the scalp. Two days later the infant died.

Histopathologic Examination. On the left in Figure 63 the wall of a bronchiole lined by pseudostratified cylindrical epithelium can be seen. In the center there is a vessel, the walls of which are heavily infiltrated by polymorphonuclear leukocytes. The lumen is partially thrombosed (H & E, 375×).

There were numerous bronchopneumonic and hemorrhagic foci in both lungs, accompanied by fibrinopurulent pleuritis. Cultures of lung tissue resulted in the isolation of many colonies of *Klebsiella pneumoniae.*

This was a case of myelomeningocele with postoperative hydrocephalus, sepsis, and multiple foci of *Klebsiella pneumoniae* infection. There was also unilateral renal agenesis.

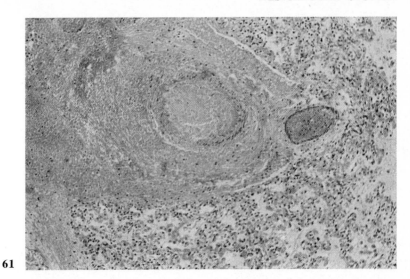

61

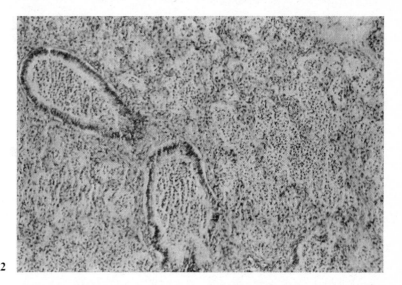

62

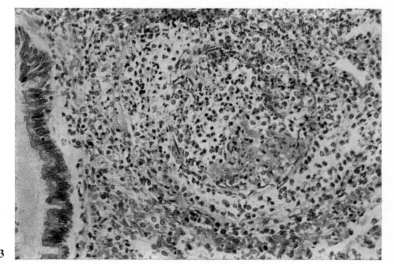

63

64
LISTERIA PNEUMONIA

Male weighing 1,200 gm. Gestational age, 30 weeks. Born by vertex presentation after 5 hour labor. Apgar score 3 at 1 minute after delivery. Resuscitation by means of intubation and oxygen therapy.

On admission 2 hours after birth the general condition was poor; there was decreased muscle tone, with slow and muffled heart beat, difficult respiration, and deep generalized cyanosis. Dextrose and bicarbonate infusion was started. Bouts of apnea appeared, and death occurred within 1 hour.

Histopathologic Examination. Figure 64 shows a granulomatoid inflammatory focus in the vicinity of a respiratory bronchiole. The exudate is composed predominantly of mononuclear leukocytes. A Levaditi stain demonstrated the presence of argyrophilic, gram-positive pleomorphic organisms (H & E, 375×). Similar foci were encountered in the liver and kidney (Fig. 196).

Other autopsy findings were subpleural petechiae and extensive subtentorial and intraventricular hemorrhage. It was suspected that the infection might have been caused by aspiration of contaminated amniotic fluid. The presence of exudate in the bronchioles and of predominantly peribronchial granulomas would seem to confirm that impression.

65
NECROTIZING PNEUMONIA

Female weighing 2,950 gm. Gestational age, 38 weeks. Admitted 3 minutes after birth.

Examination showed an anencephalic but active infant, good skin color and response to stimuli. Placed in incubator. In a few hours respiratory failure began, and studies revealed mixed metabolic and respiratory acidosis. Chest x-ray showed extensive atelectasis and an infiltrative pattern in the right lung field, suggestive of aspiration. Death occurred at 5 days of age.

Histopathologic Examination. In the upper portion of Figure 65 a large area of necrosis with loss of the normal architecture of the lung

is observed. The alveolar septa are destroyed, and there are abundant nuclear remnants. The neighboring parenchyma shows intraalveolar granulocytic and macrophagic reaction (H & E, 375×).

Other areas were emphysematous. In addition to anencephaly there was adrenal hypoplasia (combined weight 1.09 gm), and there were renal anomalies (Fig. 180).

66/67
PULMONARY STAPHYLOCOCCAL INFECTION

Ten day old male weighing 3,400 gm with a 3 day history of fever, cough, mild cyanosis, and respiratory difficulty.

X-rays showed nodular densities suggestive of bronchopneumonia, predominantly on the right. pH 7.21, pCO_2 68 mm Hg, BE −2 mEq/L.

Intensive antibiotic therapy was instituted, but the respiratory insufficiency increased. Hemogram showed marked shift to the left.

Repeated chest x-ray 48 hours later showed left pneumothorax with marked mediastinal shift and nodular pneumonic consolidation in the right lung field. Thoracentesis yielded 15 ml of purulent fluid. Culture yielded very numerous colonies of *Staphylococcus* sensitive to various antibiotics.

Further radiographic studies showed progression of the changes in the lung and increased pleural effusion in spite of intensive treatment. A drain was inserted in the left side of the chest. Bouts of cyanosis recurred. One of them culiminated in death 10 days after admission.

Histopathologic Examination. Microscopic sections of the lung showed necrotizing fibrinopurulent pleuritis and bronchopneumonic foci with abscess formation and cavitation.

Figure 66 represents the wall of one of the cavities, consisting of a solid collection of polymorphonuclear leukocytes (H & E, 187.5×).

More peripherally the process shows a tendency to fibrosis of the alveolar walls and the alveolar lining cells have become cuboidal, irregular, and swollen. Within the air spaces there are fibrinopurulent plugs with incipient organization (Fig. 67, H & E, 375×).

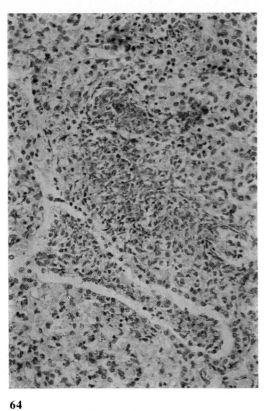

64

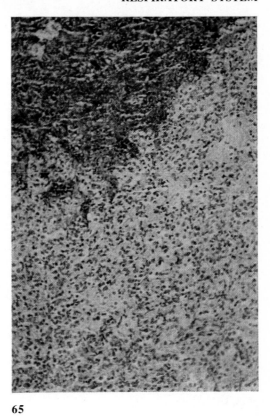

65

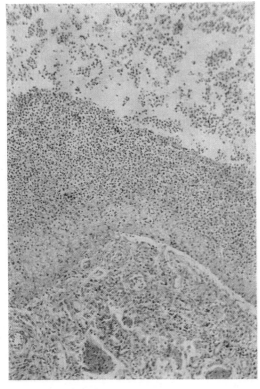

66

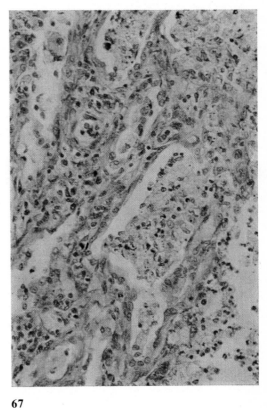

67

68/69/70
ACUTE NECROTIZING PLEURITIS WITH "DISSECTING PNEUMONIA"

Male weighing 1,600 gm. Gestational age, 30 weeks. Twin birth with cephalic presentation. Rupture of membranes 3 hours prior to delivery. Admitted at 6 hours of life, having been transported in unsanitary conditions.

Physical examination on admission, normal. Twenty-four hours later the general condition was poor; generalized hypotonia, circulatory collapse, and respiratory distress. Studies showed metabolic acidosis. Death occurred an hour later.

Histopathologic Examination. Under low magnification the visceral pleura appears thickened by virtue of an exudate with scanty leukocytic reaction (Fig. 68, H & E, 187.5×).

Gram stain brings out an accumulation of gram-positive organisms at this level (Fig. 69, 375×).

In other areas both the visceral pleura and the interlobular connective tissue septa appear thickened; here granulocytic infiltration is striking. Note the absence of exudate within the adjoining alveoli, whose septa are moderately congested (Fig. 70, H & E, 187.5×).

71
FOCAL EOSINOPHILIC INFLAMMATION WITH GIANT CELLS (IN INTERLOBULAR SEPTUM)

Male weighing 1,300 gm. Unknown gestational age. Admitted at 4 hours of life. Poor general condition, loss of muscle tone, generalized cyanosis, slow heart beat. X-rays taken at 12 hours of age were compatible with the diagnosis of hyaline membrane disease. pH 7.15, pCO_2 65 mm Hg, BE −8 mEq/L. Bicarbonate solution given to correct acidosis. Death at 16 hours.

Histopathologic Examination. Figure 71 shows an interlobular septum with a granulomatous lesion consisting of multinucleated giant cells clustered around hyaline foci and surrounded by inflammatory cells, predominantly eosinophiles (H & E, 375×).

The interpretation of this lesion is difficult. It may be related to lymphatic transport of aspirated foreign matter. In cases of severe hypoxia, interstitial eosinophilic infiltrates are often accompanied by foci of extramedullary hematopoiesis; such is not the case here.

This was an instance of pulmonary atelectasis with scanty hyaline membranes and moderate pulmonary immaturity. There were also hemorrhages in the brain and thymus.

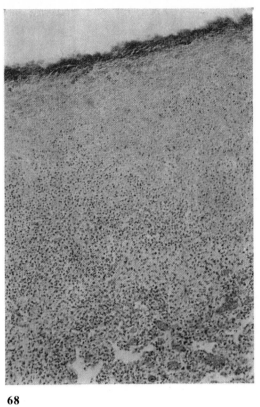

68

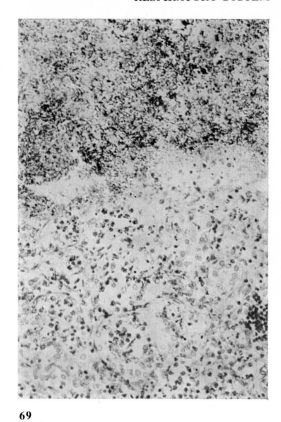

69

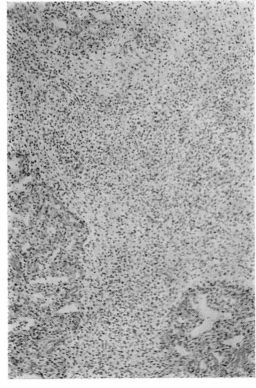

70

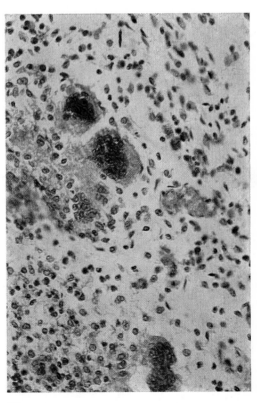

71

72/73
MONOCYTIC PNEUMONIA

Full-term male weighing 3,300 gm. At 17 days of age he was admitted for respiratory difficulty and cyanosis precipitated by crying. Body weight 2,700 gm. Symptoms were aggravated by feeding.

Chest x-ray revealed air-filled cavities in the left hemithorax. Barium enema revealed a diaphragmatic hernia, which was then corrected surgically. A few days later bouts of vomiting occurred. Further radiographic studies demonstrated a hiatal hernia. Diarrheic stools were cultured and yielded colonies of enteropathogenic *E. coli,* type O:55/B:5. Blood culture was negative. Vomiting persisted and the nutritional state deteriorated. There was progressive respiratory insufficiency. pH 7.3, pCO_2 65 mm Hg, BE +1 mEq/L.

Prolonged periods of apnea necessitated intubation and assisted respiration. Chest x-ray was suggestive of interstitial pneumonia.

Death supervened at 38 days of life.

Histopathologic Examination. In contrast to the granulocytic nature of the usual bacterial bronchopneumonia, this is conspicuous for the exclusively monocytic exudate in all alveoli. The septa exhibit congestion and partial destruction but lack interstitial infiltration (Fig. 72, H & E, 375×).

In some fields the alveolar exudate is accompanied by necrotic debris (Fig. 73, H & E, 375×).

Culture of the lung grew many colonies of *E. coli. E. coli* can also, on occasion, produce interstitial pneumonitis, as well as monocytic pneumonia such as this.

74/75
"HEART FAILURE" CELLS IN THE LUNG

Male weighing 2,740 gm. Gestational age, 40 weeks. Spontaneous delivery.

Admitted at 5 days of life because of respiratory difficulty with whining. There was generalized cyanosis, rapid breathing, and slight hepatomegaly. Respiratory acidosis. pH 7.32, pCO_2 55 mm Hg. BE−1 mEq/L.

X-rays: Uniform cardiac enlargement. Special cardiologic studies permitted a diagnosis of preductal coarctation and hypoplasia of the two left chambers. After treatment for cardiac failure the respiratory insufficiency persisted.

At 36 days of life, the infant died.

Histopathologic Examination. Figure 74 shows moderate collapse and septal congestion. The alveolar spaces are filled with desquamated phagocytic alveolar cells laden with hemosiderin ("heart failure" cells) that appear in the form of irregular, brownish corpuscles (H & E, 600×). The blue color assumed by the pigment when stained by the Perls method proves that iron is one of the components (Fig. 75, 375×). A positive reaction with PAS indicates the presence of a hydrocarbon in the hemosiderin pigment.

A preductal coarctation from which the left subclavian artery arose was demonstrated at autopsy.

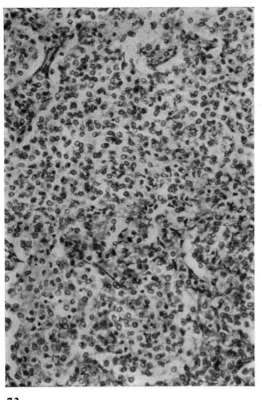

72

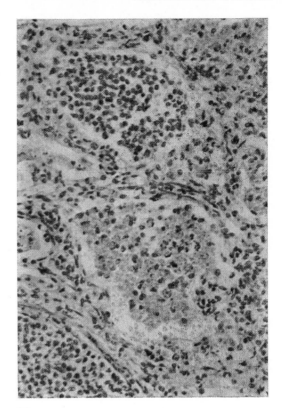

73

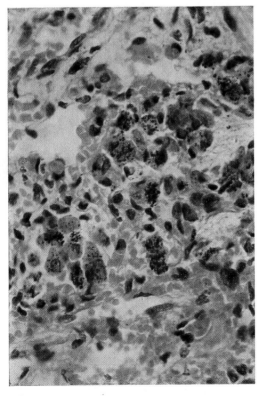

74

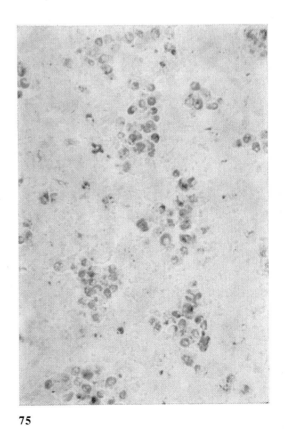

75

76
INTERSTITIAL PNEUMONIA WITH HYALINE MEMBRANE

Thirty day old female weighing 4,300 gm. Two day history of increasing respiratory difficulty. Died at the moment of admission.

Histopathologic Examination. Figure 76 shows a pattern of interstitial pneumonia with hyaline membranes and atelectasis. The alveolar septa appear thickened, partly because of alveolar collapse and partly because of inflammatory round cell infiltration. There is no cellular exudate within the alveolar spaces, the walls of which are lined by thick hyaline membranes (H & E, 187.5×).

There were also small inflammatory foci in the myocardium and in the liver; the latter showed fatty metamorphosis. Stains for bacteria and postmortem cultures were negative. These facts, together with the absence of gastrointestinal symptoms and the aforementioned microscopic findings led to diagnosis of a probably viral process.

77
INTERSTITIAL PNEUMONIA

Thirteen day old male weighing 3,100 gm. Admitted because of severe pyuria.

Hyperchloremic acidosis. Urea 1.66 gm/L. Urine culture: 302,000 colonies per milliliter of urine, identified as *E. coli*. Moderate respiratory distress became more severe within hours. pH 7.23, pCO_2 36 mm Hg, BE −13 mEq/L, chloride 126 mEq/L. Death occurred 3 days after admission.

Histopathologic Examination. Sections of the lung demonstrate the absence of exudate within the air spaces, which are markedly dilated. There are many lymphocytes in the greatly thickened alveolar septa. In some areas the picture is less pure and there are desquamated alveolar cells and large mononuclear cells in the alveolar spaces, though no phagocytosis is seen (H & E, 187.5×).

The autopsy revealed acute pyelonephritis.

78/79
CYTOMEGALIC INTERSTITIAL PNEUMONIA

Female weighing 1,500 gm. Unknown gestational age. Admitted at 24 hours of age in respiratory distress, with mixed metabolic and respiratory acidosis.

The clinical course was good until the thirtieth day of life, when gastroenteritis, metabolic acidosis, and a gluteal abscess developed. Culture of feces was negative, but from the abscess a gram-negative organism was grown. There were mild signs of respiratory difficulty, but the chest x-rays were not remarkable. There was no liver or spleen enlargement, nor were there any petechiae. Nutrition declined, and the general condition indicated sepsis.

Death occurred 45 days after birth.

Histopathologic Examination. Section of the lung shows a large number of alveolar lining cells with cytomegalic transformation, some desquamated into alveolar spaces (Fig. 78, H & E, 375×).

With greater magnification the cytomegalic cells are seen to contain large basophilic inclusion bodies within their nuclei, each surrounded by a clear halo ("bird's eye cells"). There is basophilic stippling of the cytoplasm. Conspicuous septal round cell infiltration and capillary engorgement are seen as well as intraalveolar hemorrhage (Fig. 78, H & E, 600×).

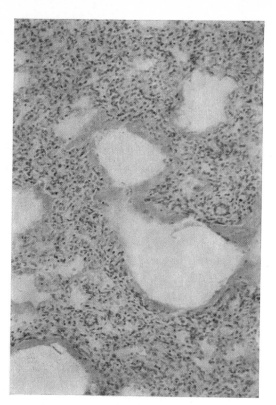

76

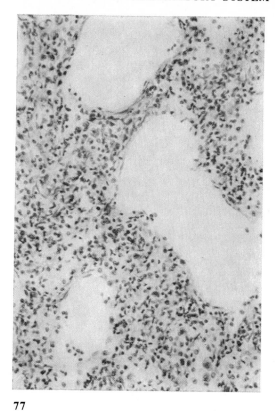

77

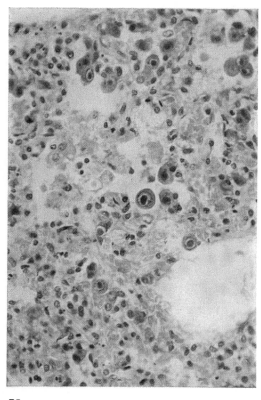

78

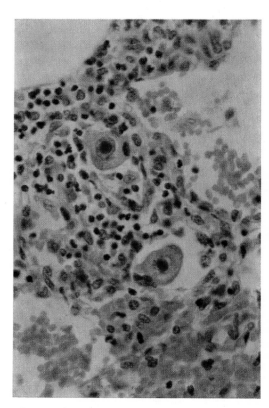

79

80/81
CANDIDA ALBICANS BRONCHOPNEUMONIA

Full-term male weighing 2,850 gm, admitted 18 hours after birth because of jaundice. Hematologic studies showed anti-A isoimmunization. Bilirubinemia, 14.5 mg/100 ml. Exchange transfusion with type O Rh negative blood was performed by the umbilical route.

Clinical course was satisfactory. Discharged in 2 weeks. Six days later he was admitted with diarrhea and dehydration, thrush, poor general condition, and respiratory difficulty. pH on admission 6.82. Two hours later he had a tonic-clonic convulsion.

(At home he had been fed hyperconcentrated milk, and sanitary conditions had been inadequate.)

Although treated for acidosis, he went into peripheral collapse and died 6 hours later.

Histopathologic Examination. The lungs show disseminated pneumonic foci, with abundant collections of granulocytes in the alveoli. Many hyphae and spores of *Candida* appear red with PAS stain (Fig. 80, 375×).

Within the wall of a bronchus, Gomori's methenamine silver method brings out septate filaments representing hyphae of *Candida* as well as small rounded bodies representing blastospores (Fig. 81, 600×).

Other findings: Left temporal subarachnoid hemorrhage, left occipital intracerebral hemorrhage, and focal renal cortical hemorrhages.

82/83
BACTERIAL AND MYCOTIC PNEUMONIA

Female weighing 1,420 gm. Cephalic delivery. Apgar score 6 at birth. Admitted at 1 hour with respiratory difficulty, cyanosis, and loss of tone. pH 7.20, pCO_2 61 mm Hg, BE −11.5 mEq/L.

She was placed in an incubator and given 10 per cent dextrose and $1/6$ M bicarbonate. For a few days she improved, and the intravenous infusion was discontinued.

Chest x-rays showed moderate confluent nodular densities. There were no signs to indicate hyaline membrane disease. Her respiratory condition improved, and feedings by nasogastric tube replaced the intravenous infusion. Feeding was not well tolerated, and she regurgitated frequently. At the age of 17 days she took a sudden turn for the worse with respiratory and metabolic acidosis. pH 7.24, pCO_2 52.5 mm Hg, BE −5 mEq/L.

Respiratory insufficiency increased, and x-rays showed diffuse densities in both lungs. Death occurred 2 days later.

Histopathologic Examination. There was extensive bilateral bronchopneumonia. Gram stain (Fig. 82) shows abundant colonies of bacteria both gram-negative and gram-positive, as well as the septate filaments and spores of *Candida*, demonstrable also by the methenamine silver method of Gomori (Fig. 83, 600×).

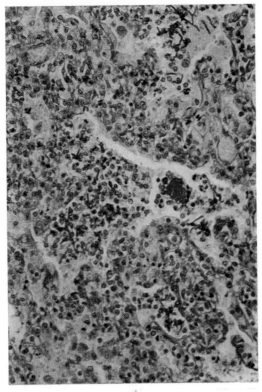

80

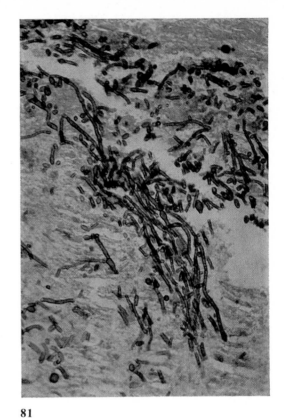

81

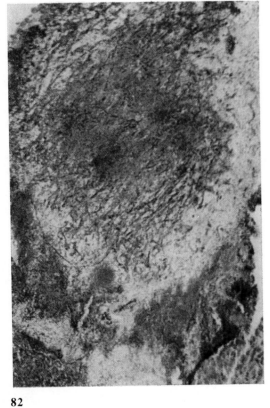

82

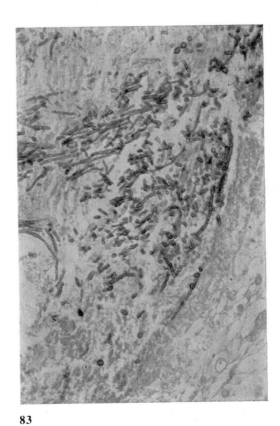

83

84/85/86
INTERSTITIAL PLASMA CELL PNEUMONIA (PNEUMOCYSTIS CARINII)

Forty-five day old male weighing 2,300 gm, admitted in marasmus, with grayish pallor, dehydration, and gastroenteritis.

He was a 2,000 gm premature at birth and was hospitalized for 12 days for that reason, but appeared in good health upon discharge. Ten days later he developed diarrhea, dehydration, and metabolic acidosis and was readmitted. He remained in the hospital for several days but gained no weight.

On that occasion x-rays showed right apical emphysema and superior mediastinal shift to the left; this was interpreted as moderate atelectasis.

Discharged in good nutritional state, he again developed diarrhea, lost weight, and presented some respiratory difficulty, all of which led to his last admission.

Acid-base balance: pH 7.33, pCO_2 48.5 mm Hg, BE −2 mEq/L. Culture of feces grew type O:111/B:4 pathogenic *E. coli*.

The dehydration was corrected, and acid-base values and electrolytes returned to normal, but there was no nutritional improvement, and respiratory insufficiency continued, culminating in death 10 days after admission.

Histopathologic Examination. Under low magnification the striking feature is filling of alveoli with an eosinophilic exudate. The alveolar septa show inflammatory infiltration (Fig. 84, H & E, 187.5 ×).

With greater magnification the exudate exhibits a characteristically foamy appearance, and cystic, refringent structures can be discerned, with minute basophilic granules at their centers. The septal infiltration consists mainly of plasma cells. The alveolar epithelium is somewhat swollen (Fig. 85, H & E, 600×).

Methenamine silver stains establish the fact that the argyrophilic corpuscles are *Pneumocystis carinii* (Fig. 86, Gomori, 600 ×).

87
PNEUMOCYSTIS CARINII PNEUMONIA WITH SCANTY SEPTAL INFILTRATION

Two month old male, premature birth, 2,000 gm weight at birth. On admission he weighed 2,800 gm. History of diarrhea for 1 month, with negative stool cultures. Bilateral suppurative otitis media. General condition, emaciated. Progressive respiratory insufficiency. Negative blood culture, negative urine culture. Exudate from the ear positive for *Streptococcus viridans*. Hematocrit 24 per cent. Hemoglobin 6.5 gm/100 ml. Leukocytes 4,300. Total protein 4.6 gm/100 ml, γ-globulin 3.89 mg/100 ml. Platelets 85,000/cu mm. Chest x-ray revealed scattered nodular densities and consolidation in the right upper lobe. Progressive respiratory insufficiency eventuated in death one month later. Tracheal exudate negative for *Pneumocystis carinii*. Probable diagnosis: *Pneumocystis* pneumonia in a child with immunodeficiency.

Histopathologic Examination. The alveolar spaces are filled with a foamy exudate in which methenamine silver stain demonstrated the presence of *Pneumocystis carinii*. There is hardly any round cell infiltration of the septa (H & E, 375×).

At autopsy there was thymic dysplasia with depletion of lymphoid structures.

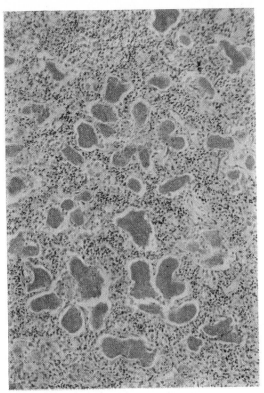

84

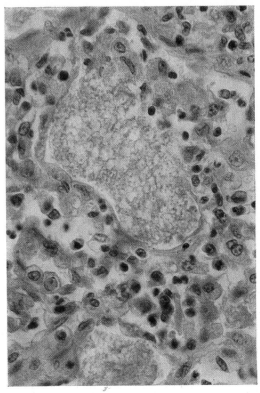

85

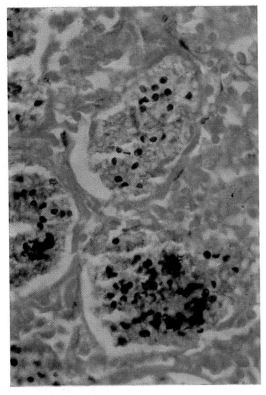

86

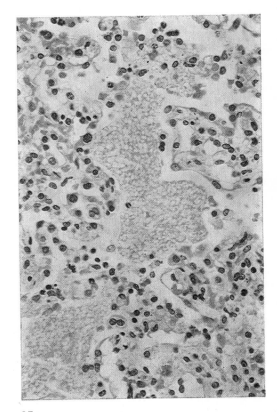

87

88
CONGENITAL CYSTIC LYMPHANGIECTASIA

One month old male weighing 3,100 gm, admitted for respiratory insufficiency with flaring of the nostrils, inspiratory retraction and signs of peripheral collapse, whining on expiration, cold extremities, and generalized hypotonia. X-rays showed consolidation in the lower portion of the right lung field and fine reticular shadows in both lungs.

pH 7.27, pCO_2 57 mm Hg, BE −2 mEq/L. Culture of gastric contents was negative.

The course was rapidly downhill; respiratory difficulty increased; the heart became uniformly enlarged, and the infant died in 30 hours.

Histopathologic Examination. In addition to bronchiolitis and hyaline membrane formation, there were lesions of congenital cystic lymphangiectasia. The interlobular septa were widened because of the marked cystic dilatation of lymphatics, each lined by delicate and ostensibly normal endothelium. In contradistinction to a true neoplastic lymphangioma, there are no lymphoid nodules in the stroma nor is there proliferation of the vascular endothelium. Also lacking is the muscular hyperplasia found in acquired obstructive lymphangiectasia (H & E, 60×). Pulmonary lymphangiectasia is found in cases of congenital absence of the spleen and is common in hyaline membrane disease.

89
CONGENITAL LOBAR EMPHYSEMA

One month old male, admitted in severe respiratory distress, weighing 3,960 gm on admission. After a difficult delivery he exhibited deep cyanosis that necessitated resuscitation.

From the first days of life he experienced respiratory difficulty and cyanotic episodes brought about by crying or coughing.

Chest x-rays showed marked emphysema over the entire right lung field, with displacement of the mediastinum into the opposite lung field. Bronchogram demonstrated enormous overaeration of the right upper lobe and collapse of the middle and lower lobes. Acid-base balance studies: pH 7.13, pCO_2 57.5 mm Hg, BE −12.2 mEq/L, pO_2 54 mm Hg, pO_2 in 100 per cent oxygen 120 mm Hg, and hemoglobin saturation 135 per cent.

Diagnosis of congenital lobar emphysema was made, and a right upper lobectomy was carried out. The postoperative course was good, and the child was discharged 1 month later.

Histopathologic Examination. The resected specimen showed very marked dilatation of alveolar atria and alveoli, with ample confluence of air spaces (H & E, 187.5×). [This lesion usually involves an upper lobe.]

Congenital lobar emphysema is a type of rapidly developing regional emphysema peculiar to the newborn and infant. In about half the cases there are no changes in the corresponding bronchus; if there are, it is usually hypoplasia of bronchial cartilage or the presence of an aberrant vessel.

90/91
CYSTIC ADENOMATOID MALFORMATION OF THE LUNG

Full-term female weighing 3,030 gm. Admitted at 3 days of age because of subcostal retraction, tympanitic percussion note in the left hemithorax, displacement of heart sounds to the right, and absence of breath sounds in the left side of the chest. pH 7.41, pCO_2 35 mm Hg, BE −2 mEq/L.

Chest films showed a rounded, very radiolucent image in the left basal area, which eventually depressed the diaphragm and displaced the lung upward, collapsing it. Tomograms showed no bifurcation of the left bronchus and did not show signs of bronchial distortion.

The clinical diagnosis was "probable left lower lobe lobar emphysema." The location, unusual for that entity, left open the possibility of a bronchial cyst. A left thoracotomy was performed. A series of ampullary formations, as much as 2 to 3 cm in diameter, were seen in the left lower lobe. A lobectomy was performed.

The child was discharged fully recovered 25 days later.

Histopathologic Examination. The specimen consisted of a cystic structure composed of multiple irregular cavities. The cysts were lined by bronchial mucosa with pseudopapillary formations (Fig. 90, H & E, 60×). With greater magnification an outer smooth muscle layer can be recognized; the lining is of cylindrical epithelium, ciliated in places (Fig. 91, H & E, 375×). There were no hyaline cartilage plates.

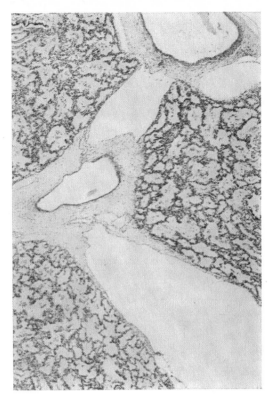

88

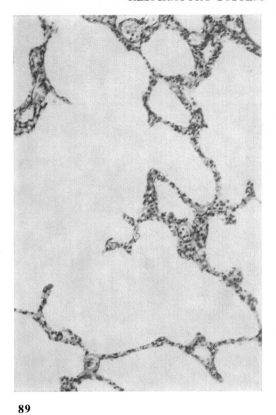

89

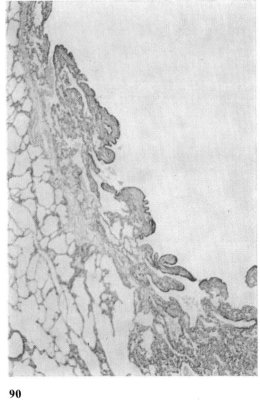

90

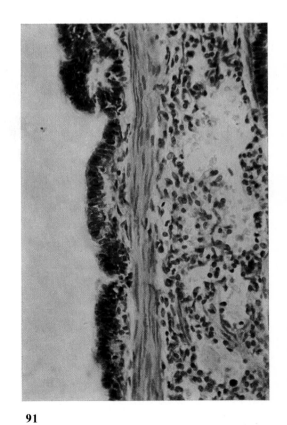

91

92/93
CONGENITAL CYSTIC BRONCHIOLECTASIS

Morphologically intersexual newborn weighing 2,000 gm. Gestational age, 30 weeks; admitted 24 hours after birth because of imperforate anus, respiratory difficulty, poor general condition, and cyanosis. Implantation of the ears was low.

Died 12 hours later in respiratory failure with cyanosis and marked hypotonia.

Histopathologic Examination. Figure 92 shows a number of irregular cystic structures (H & E, 187.5×).

With greater magnification the lining epithelium can be seen to be cylindrical and ciliated. The alveoli have a glandular appearance and show hemorrhagic infiltration of the septa (Fig. 93, H & E, 375×).

As is usual in this type of congenital cystic anomaly of the lung, only one lobe was affected, in this case the right lower lobe.

Other malformations were noted at autopsy: (a) agenesis of the bladder; (b) agenesis of the right kidney and ureter; (c) hypoplasia-dysplasia of the left kidney with termination of the corresponding ureter at the base of the penis; (d) location of testicles at the level of the inguinal canals; and (e) hypospadias.

94/95
CYSTIC FIBROSIS OF THE PANCREAS, PULMONARY INVOLVEMENT

Female weighing 3,900 gm. Gestational age, 40 weeks. Admitted at 24 hours of life with symptoms of intestinal obstruction. The diagnosis was meconium ileus, and surgery was performed the same day. Sixty-four centimeters of dilated bowel was resected. The infant died of complications of the surgical procedure 18 days later.

Histopathologic Examination. Figure 94 shows bronchiolectasis with purulent bronchiolitis in adjacent parenchyma and a large area of emphysema. There were many areas of atelectasis attributable to intrinsic bronchiolar obstruction (Masson, 60×).

In the trachea the glandular acini and excretory ducts were distended with mucus (Fig. 95, PAS, 375×).

Histologic study of the pancreas shows cystic transformation of most of the acini, their lumina filled with mucoid material, and interstitial fibrosis (Fig. 236). Similarly, there was cystic dilatation of Brunner's glands. Purulent peritonitis was present with perihepatitis and perisplenitis.

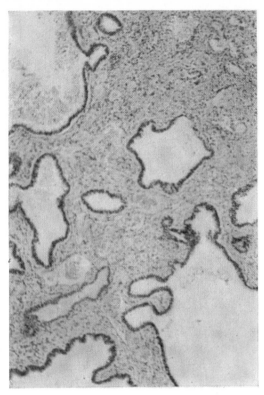

92

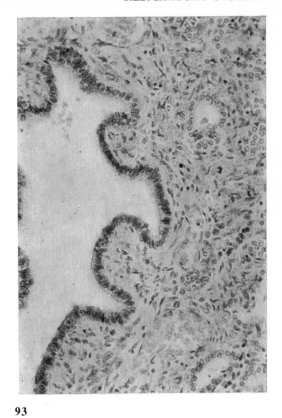

93

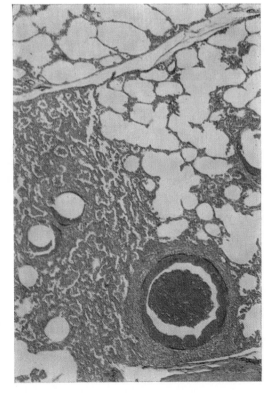

94

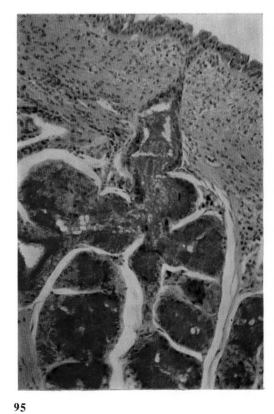

95

PULMONARY THROMBOSES. DISSEMINATED INTRAVASCULAR COAGULOPATHY

Male weighing 2,700 gm. Gestational age, 39 weeks. Cephalic delivery after 6 hours' labor. Rupture of membranes 2 days before.

Admitted at 30 hours of life in poor general condition and respiratory distress. At birth, energetic resuscitative measures had been employed, including aspiration, intubation, and administration of oxygen.

Respiratory acidosis with pH 7.16, pCO_2 65 mm Hg, BE -9 mEq/L. Dextrose solution with 1 M bicarbonate and antibiotics was given.

Culture of gastric contents was negative. Culture of pharyngeal mucus yielded innumerable colonies of *Klebsiella pneumoniae*. Chest films showed a pattern consistent with aspiration pneumonia. Subsequent course was stormy, punctuated by bouts of apnea and intense cyanosis in spite of oxygen therapy.

Death supervened at 54 hours of life.

Histopathologic Examination. Figure 96 shows a dilated venule filled with an adherent fibrino-leukocytic thrombus. There were also extensive bronchopneumonic foci alternating with areas of atelectasis (H & E, 375×).

Figure 97 illustrates intracapillary hyaline pulmonary thrombi. This section is from a full-term newborn who died at 20 hours of age with cyanosis and respiratory failure. There was no concomitant septic syndrome, but similar thrombi were seen in the capillaries and other small vessels of the myocardium, brain, and intestinal submucosa (H & E, 375×).

Pulmonary arterial and venous thrombosis is often seen in bronchopneumonic, suppurative, and necrotizing processes.

In this case there was extensive pulmonary atelectasis and meningeal hemorrhagic infiltration. Coagulation studies were not available.

SEPTIC PULMONARY THROMBUS

Male weighing 1,750 gm. Unknown gestational age. Admitted at 2 hours of life. Physical examination was normal, and the child was discharged at 18 days of age with a weight of 2,500 gm. A week later he was readmitted with severe diarrhea, in poor general condition, with grayish pallor, irritability, mild dehydration, and 2 fingerbreadth hepatomegaly. Acid-base studies showed: pH 7.09, pCO_2 40 mm Hg, BE -17 mEq/L. The microhematocrit was 37 per cent. Sodium 136 mEq/L, chloride 85 mEq/L. Fecal culture produced type 0111:K58(B4) *E. coli* and numerous colonies of *Candida*.

Despite antibiotic treatment and other measures, the course was unfavorable. Frank respiratory insufficiency appeared. Chest radiographs showed scattered densities. Blood culture grew *Klebsiella pneumoniae* very sensitive to gentamicin. Diarrhea persisted; breathing did not improve, and hemorrhagic phenomena appeared. Death followed 15 days after admission.

Histopathologic Examination. Figure 98 shows, as a central focus of sepsis, a pulmonary vein containing a polypoid parietal thrombus covered by a fibrinous layer in which there is a nest of leukocytes (H & E, 187.5×). Special stains demonstrated the presence of *Candida*.

At autopsy there was bilateral pneumonia with multiple foci of gram-negative organisms identified as *Klebsiella* by culture with necrotizing hemorrhagic enteritis, and *Candida* granulomas in the lung, intestine, adrenals, and liver.

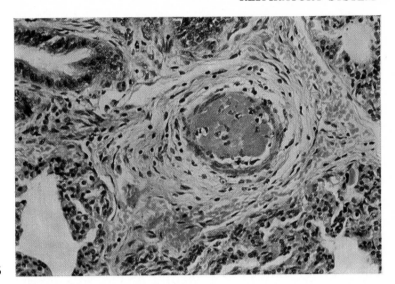

96

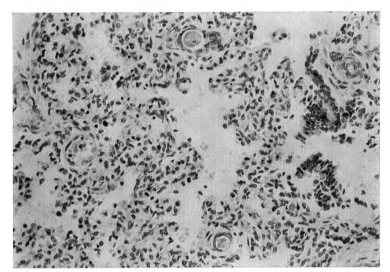

97

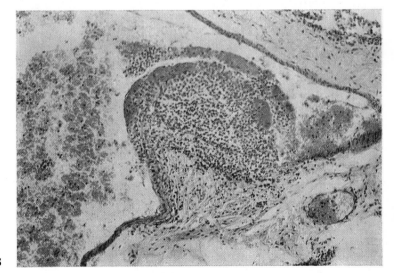

98

WILSON-MIKITY SYNDROME

Male weighing 1,220 gm. Gestational age, 31 weeks. Apgar score 10.

Admitted 3 hours after delivery. Examination revealed that the infant had Down's syndrome. The first 19 days of life were uneventful. At that point, respiratory symptoms began and increased gradually thereafter.

Chest films showed bilateral infiltration in the form of a coarse reticular pattern circumscribing small cystic spaces about 2 mm in diameter. This created a bizarre appearance quite characteristic of the early phases of the Wilson-Mikity syndrome.

There was little change during the next 20 days, but then the patient's respiratory difficulties worsened. Radiographically, the reticular pattern seemed to regress, and basal emphysema became more obvious. In addition, parahilar infiltration appeared; the impression was that the patient was in the second phase of the disease.

Respiratory acidosis: pH 7.19, pCO_2 63 mm Hg, BE -6.5 mEq/L.

Continuous progression of the respiratory difficulty required confinement in an incubator with oxygen administration. When the patient was 60 days of age the respiratory problem was still apparent.

In spite of 1 M bicarbonate infusion and oxygen, the values were: pH 7.22, pCO_2 60 mm Hg, arterial pO_2 46 mm Hg in 100 per cent oxygen, BE -3 mEq/L.

The patient's dyspnea worsened and his acidosis increased: pH 6.85, pCO_2 120 mm Hg, BE -14 mEq/L. He died at the age of 65 days.

Histopathologic Examination. Microscopic examination of the lungs showed two basic types of lesions, irregularly distributed: (a) wide areas of emphysema with rupture of alveolar septa and formation of large air spaces (Fig. 99, Masson, 60×); and (b) moderate interstitial pulmonary fibrosis represented in Figure 100 by thickening of alveolar septa due to the presence of connective tissue fibers, which stain green with trichrome stain (Masson, 375×). There is no inflammatory infiltrate or exudate. There were no other findings of interest.

PULMONARY DYSMATURITY

Male weighing 750 gm. Gestational age, 25 weeks. Delivery in cephalic presentation 8 days after the rupture of the membranes. Apgar score 1 at birth, requiring resuscitation. Admitted 10 hours after birth with signs of respiratory insufficiency and evidence of marked immaturity. Cultures of gastric contents, meconium, pharyngeal secretions, and umbilical vein blood were all negative. Prophylactic antibiotic treatment was started. Feeding was difficult. Mixed acidosis: pH 7.19, pCO_2 56 mm Hg, BE -9.5, mEq/L. Microhematocrit 64 per cent. Platelets 86,000/cu mm. For 20 days poor general condition continued with periods of acidosis in spite of corrective bicarbonate therapy. The respiratory syndrome was stable. The patient had intermittent diarrhea, but stool cultures were negative. At 28 days of life the infant died with moderate sclerema. He had failed to gain weight. Several chest films during the course of his illness had shown mild atelectasis, but no definite diagnosis was made.

Histopathologic Examination. Figure 101 shows markedly thickened alveolar septa without inflammatory infiltration (H & E, 375×). Trichrome stains demonstrated moderate septal fibrosis. In Figure 102 considerable edema of the septa is apparent as well as dilated capillaries that are rather distant from the alveolar lining. There is no exudate in the air spaces (H & E, 600×). Note the similarity of this picture to Figure 30, interpreted as acquired pulmonary dysplasia probably secondary to oxygen therapy. This newborn of very low birth weight, who lived for 28 days, required oxygen for only the first week of life. The question of the role of oxygen therapy also comes up with regard to the pathogenesis of the Wilson-Mikity syndrome.

In this case the autopsy revealed marked cerebral and renal immaturity, the latter expressed by a broad, continuous nephrogenic zone. There were no foci of hematopoiesis in the liver, although the trabeculae were thick.

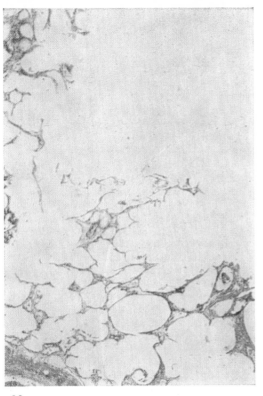

99

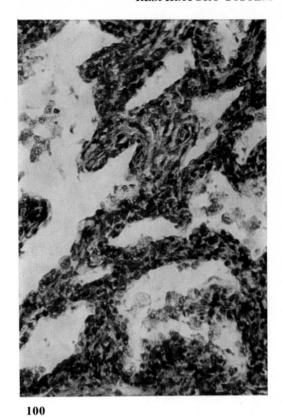

100

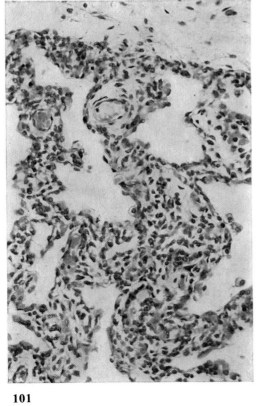

101

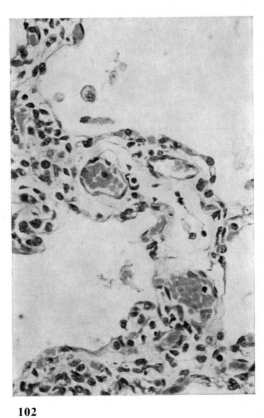

102

103
HETEROTOPIC BRAIN TISSUE IN THE LUNG

Male weighing 2,400 gm. Gestational age, 31 weeks. Cephalic delivery. Apgar score 5 at birth. On examination, there was anencephaly with a minute encephalic nodule without any bony covering, generalized hypotonia, and gasping respirations. Died in 4 hours.

Histopathologic Examination. Figure 103 represents a section of lung at the edge of a lobe. This triangular zone is well demarcated from the adjacent parenchyma and is made up of a conglomerate of vessels in the midst of glial tissue (Masson, 15×). In addition to anencephaly, the autopsy showed hypoplastic dysplastic kidneys and, as is usual in such cases, adrenal hypoplasia. The lungs, also hypoplastic, weighed 12 and 14 gm.

104
BRAIN TISSUE EMBOLISM IN PULMONARY VESSEL

Male weighing 1,000 gm. Gestational age, 28 weeks. Born by cephalic presentation with Apgar score 5 at 1 minute. Admitted at 1 hour in poor general condition with marked hypotonia and obvious signs of immaturity. Arterial pH 7.06, pCO$_2$ 35.5 mm Hg, BE −18.5 mEq/L. Microhematocrit 45 per cent, total protein 3.4 gm/100 ml. Chest x-ray was noncontributory. As the plan of treatment was being considered there were frequent episodes of apnea. Death occurred at 6 hours.

Histopathologic Examination. Figure 104 shows a pulmonary arterial branch plugged by glial tissue with vessels (H & E, 187.5×). Similar embolic material was seen in other pulmonary vessels and in a branch of the renal artery. Other autopsy findings are enumerated with Figure 195.

105
HAMARTOMATOID PERIPHERAL BRONCHOPULMONARY DYSPLASIA

Male weighing 3,000 gm. Gestational age, 37 weeks. Normal delivery. Apgar score 10. Admitted at 5 hours of life because of bile-tinged vomitus and marked abdominal distention. On examination, good general condition and adequate activity, but globular, distended, and tympanitic abdomen. A nasogastric tube was passed and 150 ml of bile-stained fluid was recovered. Radiographs confirmed the clinical impression of intestinal obstruction. Laparotomy revealed multiple jejunal atresias. For the first 3 days the postoperative course was satisfactory, but then signs of gastric retention and intestinal obstruction reappeared. Chest films indicated the presence of bilateral bronchopneumonia. Surgical reexploration disclosed the existence of hemoperitoneum related to laceration of the outer coats of the terminal large bowel. Progressive respiratory failure necessitated the use of assisted respiration; death supervened at 10 days.

Histopathologic Examination. The lungs weighed 60 and 65 gm. There were roughly wedge-shaped depressions, grayish and fibrous, on the pleural surfaces, especially on the left. On section these areas were up to 7 mm in thickness. Figure 105 illustrates one of them, showing dilated, microcystic bronchioles, plaques of cartilage, and sequestered islands of pulmonary parenchyma (Masson, 60×).

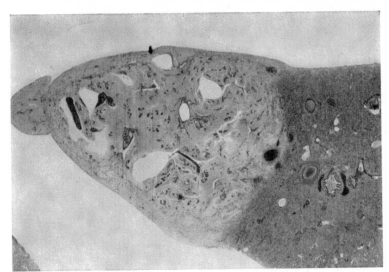

103

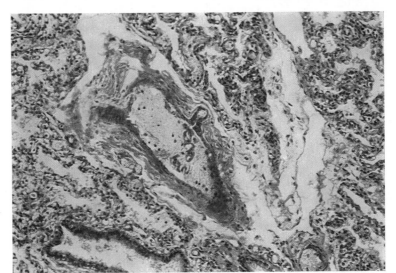

104

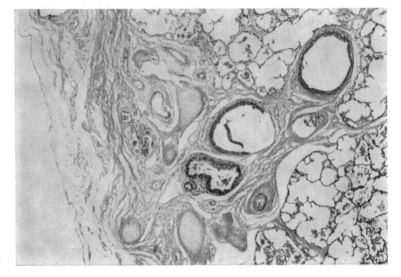

105

Heart

106
CONGENITAL PURULENT PERICARDITIS

Full-term male weighing 3,000 gm. Normal delivery. No other data available. Spontaneous cry at birth, followed by the onset of respiratory insufficiency, cyanosis, intercostal inspiratory retraction, and poor general condition. Death occurred on admission, at 2 hours of life.

Histopathologic Examination. The visceral pericardium is markedly thickened, edematous, and profusely infiltrated by granulocytes, with a lesser participation of round cells. The adjacent myocardium is normal (H & E, 375×).

Aside from moderate atelectasis, there were no other significant findings. There was no pleuritis, pneumonia, or any sign of sepsis. This brief survival leads to the supposition that the pericarditis was congenital.

107
PURULENT PERICARDITIS

Male weighing 1,250 gm. Gestational age, 29 weeks. Breech delivery. Apgar score 8 at birth.

On admission, 1 hour after birth, there was respiratory distress, which subsided within 24 hours. Good general condition was maintained until the seventh day, at which time his condition deteriorated; there were dryness of skin and mucosae, abdominal distention, and pyodermatitis. From the latter lesions a coagulase-positive *Staphylococcus* was isolated. In spite of treatment, his condition became worse. Chest x-rays demonstrated infiltrative-nodular lesions. At 28 days of age the infant died with generalized sepsis, pyodermatitis, and cutaneous abscesses.

Histopathologic Examination. The pericardium is thickened and infiltrated by an exudate consisting mainly of mononuclear cells; there are few granulocytes. On the surface there is a layer of partially organized fibrin (H & E, 375×).

Other findings included acute erosive enteritis and hepatic cholestasis. The lungs were normal.

108
FIBRINOUS PERICARDITIS

Female weighing 2,900 gm. Gestational age, 37 weeks.

Admitted at 40 hours of life because of abdominal distention and fecaloid vomiting. Radiologic studies indicated intestinal obstruction. The existence of an annular pancreas also determined at surgery. A gastrostomy was instituted, and an indwelling tube was left in place. Twenty-four hours later cardiorespiratory arrest occurred but was resolved by resuscitation. pH 7.29, pCO$_2$ 46.5 mm Hg, BE −4.5 mEq/L. These deviations were corrected. Three days later respiratory inadequacy increased and the acid-base balance showed pH 7.40, pCO$_2$ 64 mm Hg, BE +9.5 mEq/L.

Manifestations of general sepsis, sclerema, apnea, and cyanosis supervened; death occurred 5 days after surgery.

Histopathologic Examination. The visceral pericardium is thickened and shows a mild degree of polymorphonuclear infiltration. The surface is covered by a band of fibrin with villous or pseudopapillary formations. There are multiple bacterial colonies, especially on the free surfaces. The mesothelial cells of the pericardium are swollen (H & E, 375×). There was also purulent mediastinitis.

109
HETEROTOPIC HEMATOPOIESIS IN VISCERAL PERICARDIUM

Male weighing 1,650 gm. Gestational age, 32 weeks. Cephalic delivery 48 hours after rupture of membranes. Apgar score 3 at birth, requiring resuscitation.

On admission, 2 hours after birth; poor general condition, cyanosis, generalized edema, respiratory distress, and mixed acidosis. Chest films suggested hyaline membrane disease. At 7 hours there was a turn for the worse with bouts of apnea, culminating in death.

Histopathologic Examination. A circumscribed area of the pericardium showed a group of dilated capillaries in the center of a focus of elements of hematopoietic type, including numerous erythroblasts and some myeloid cells (H & E, 375×).

The localized nature and cell type distinguish this lesion from suppurative congenital pericarditis.

There was no sign of erythroblastosis nor was there any ostensible hematopoiesis in other organs.

Other autopsy findings were infratentorial and intraventricular hemorrhages, atelectasis, and hyaline membrane disease.

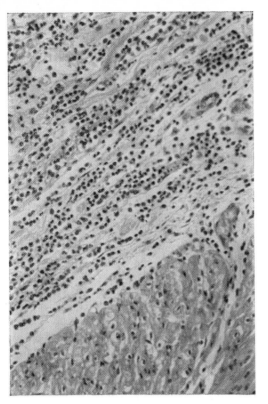

106

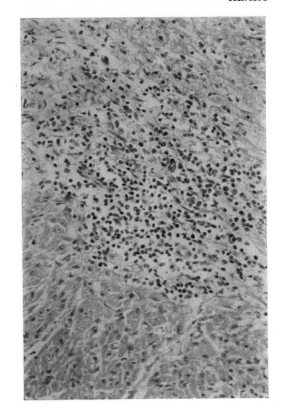

107

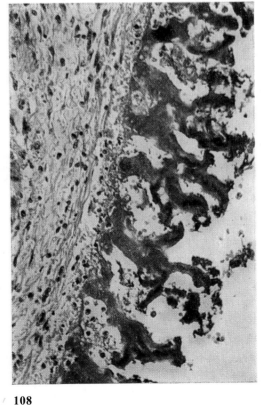

108

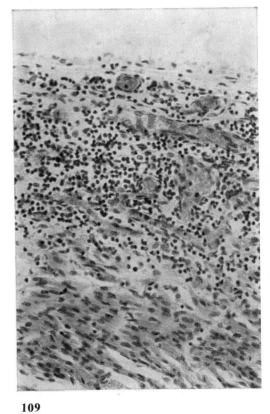

109

110/111
GRANULOMATOUS EOSINOPHILIC EPICARDITIS

Male weighing 2,800 gm. Gestational age, 40 weeks. Breech presentation. Marked cyanosis, weak cry, general loss of tone, respiratory insufficiency. Systolic murmurs in all areas, anal atresia, low implantation of ears, and clubfeet. Chest x-rays showed no changes compatible with hyaline membrane disease. Death at 2 hours.

Histopathologic Examination. In the vicinity of a blood vessel in the epicardium a granulomatous lesion can be seen. It is made up of a central necrobiotic zone containing nuclear remnants surrounded by dense eosinophilic infiltration (Fig. 110, Masson, 60×).

With greater magnification it is apparent that the infiltrate consists predominantly of mature eosinophils with a moderate number of histiocytes. There is no vascular lesion (Fig. 111, H & E, 600×).

This type of granuloma was encountered only in the epicardium; there were no lesions in other organs.

Our material includes 3 other cases of eosinophilic granulomatous epicarditis with similar morphologic characteristics. In all of them the changes were confined to the heart. There was no vasculitis or involvement of other organs. The location in the vicinity of vessels of large caliber was a striking feature. In 2 of the cases there were anomalies that were incompatible with life.

In this autopsy, in addition to anal atresia and rectourethral fistula, there was a right polycystic kidney with hypoplasia, left megaureter, right urethral atresia, and mural hyperplasia of the urinary bladder. There was a complex cardiac anomaly, comprising transposition of great vessels, single atrium, tricuspid agenesis, interventricular septal defect, and persistent ductus arteriosus. Rib development was anomalous, and there was a cartilaginous retrosymphyseal ring overlying the urethra and the rectal blind pouch.

112
SEPTIC MYOCARDITIS

Full-term male weighing 3,460 gm. Admitted at 7 days of age in poor general condition with fever, abdominal distention, diarrhea, and signs of respiratory failure. Blood culture was positive for type 111:B4 *E. coli*. Stool culture and spinal fluid were also positive for that organism. The spinal tap yielded purulent material. The organisms were sensitive to gentamicin and kanamycin. There was, however, no response to therapeutic measures. The course was unfavorable; sepsis continued, and respiratory distress increased. On the eleventh day the child died.

Histopathologic Examination. Figure 112 shows predominantly mononuclear infiltration of the myocardium; there are few granulocytes. The blue, granular clumps are bacterial colonies. There is edema separating the myocardial fibers (H & E, 375×).

Cultures from the tissues were positive for *E. coli*. Other findings included purulent meningitis and sepsis.

113
PRIMARY MYOCARDITIS

Male weighing 3,500 gm. Gestational age, 36 weeks. Apgar score 10 at birth. Normal delivery. Five days later a whining cry with rapid irregular breathing and deep cyanosis prompted admission. At that time there was jaundice; the total bilirubin was 18.6 mg/100 ml. Good general condition. pH 7.34, pCO_2 40 mm Hg, BE −4 mEq/L. Standard measures were employed. Three days later there was still rapid breathing with perioral cyanosis and pallor. pH 7.27, pCO_2 75 mm Hg, BE −1 mEq/L, hematocrit 40 per cent, total bilirubin 8.37 mg/100 ml. There was no diarrhea. In a few hours the situation grew much worse. Respirations became gasping and the heart rate slow. Death followed swiftly.

Histopathologic Examination. The heart was flabby and weighed 40 gm. Microscopically, there was a dense interstitial infiltration of the myocardium, mainly lymphocytic (H & E, 375×).

The inflammatory process was limited to the heart; no other organ was affected.

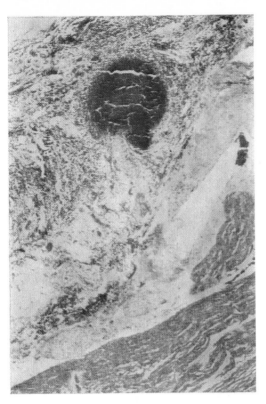

110

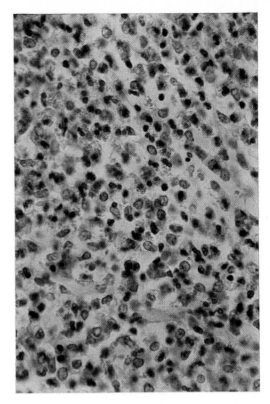

111

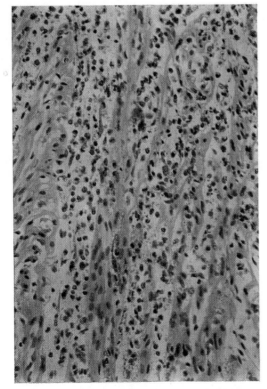

112

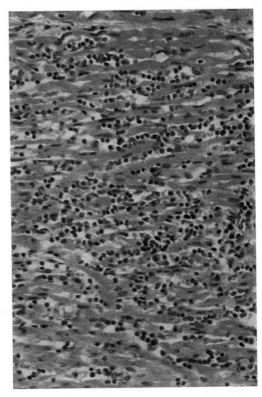

113

114
CYTOMEGALIC INCLUSION MYOCARDITIS

Male weighing 2,800 gm. Gestational age, 34 weeks. Admitted at 6 hours of life in poor general condition with severe jaundice and purpura. There was marked hepatosplenomegaly.

Isoimmunization was ruled out by means of pertinent studies. Microhematocrit 60 per cent, total bilirubin 25 mg/100 ml, indirect bilirubin 21 mg/100 ml. Exchange transfusion was carried out by the umbilical route. Jaundice persisted; bilirubin levels in succeeding hours were between 17 and 12 mg/100 ml. Eye-ground examination revealed a right papillary hemorrhage. Chest films showed cardiomegaly with a cardiothoracic index of 0.64 (normal 0.55).

Cultures of urine, meconium, and spinal fluid were negative, as was the blood culture. Repeated examinations of urine sediment revealed cells diagnostic of cytomegalic inclusion disease. Purpura increased, the general condition worsened, myoclonic seizures appeared in the extremities, blood tinged mucus was expelled by mouth, and the infant died 60 hours after admission.

Histopathologic Examination. The area shown in Figure 114 represents focal destruction of myocardial fibers. It is accompanied by interstitial edema and inflammatory infiltration. A number of "bird's eye"—type giant cells may be seen. Each contains a large intranuclear basophilic inclusion that is surrounded by a clear halo. The nuclear chromatin is marginated, and the cytoplasm is basophilic and granular (H & E, 600×).

Typical cytomegalic lesions were also seen in the lung, liver, and spleen.

115
CANDIDA MYOCARDITIS

Male weighing 3,400 gm, admitted at 13 days of life because of a strangulated right inguinal hernia. Forty-eight hours before admission he developed frequent vomiting, irritability, constipation, and a palpable right inguinal mass, with a body temperature of 104° F. On admission his general condition was poor. X-rays showed dilated intestinal loops with a few air-fluid levels. After hydration and correction of electrolyte imbalance, surgery was performed. There was abundant purulent ascites. The ileum was perforated some 3 cm above the cecum. An 8 cm segment of small bowel was bound by adhesions and had to be resected along with the right colon. A right-sided ileos-

tomy was established, and the transverse colon was brought out at the incision.

Cultures of peritoneal fluid were positive for *E. coli* and coagulase positive *Staphylococcus*. Gastric and intestinal contents were positive for *Candida albicans*.

The postoperative course was stormy; there were bouts of collapse and of respiratory and cardiac arrest, which responded to resuscitation. Twenty-five days later a definitive end-to-end anastomosis was carried out. The child's condition was generally poor; nutrition was inadequate, and stool cultures continued to be positive for *Candida* in spite of treatment. Five days after the second operation he died.

Histopathologic Examination. In the center of Figure 115 hyphae and spores of *Candida* are seen, stained black by the methenamine silver method (Gomori, 600×). Other fields showed microabscesses. The liver, lungs, and kidneys also bore abscesses and granulomas caused by *Candida*.

116
CONGENITAL TOXOPLASMOSIS WITH INVOLVEMENT OF MYOCARDIUM

Female weighing 2,480 gm. Gestational age, 32 weeks. Rupture of membranes 24 hours before delivery. Apgar score 4 at birth, necessitating resuscitation.

On admission: Poor general condition, hypotonia, lagging reflexes, left-sided microophthalmia, moderate subcostal retraction, midsystolic murmur. Chest x-ray showed cardiomegaly. Spinal tap: Grossly clear, negative culture. pH 7.26, pCO$_2$ 58 mm Hg, BE −3 mEq/L, SGOT 104 u/L, SGPT 86 u/L, LDH 290 u/L.

Cardiologic studies suggested myocarditis. Standard incubator measures, digitalization, and oxygen therapy were employed. Repeated bouts of apnea required multiple resuscitative maneuvers. Death supervened on the fifth hospital day.

Histopathologic Examination. In the center of Figure 116 a rounded, acidophilic structure is noted. It contains oval or crescent-shaped basophilic granules, representing *Toxoplasma* pseudocysts. Myocardial fibers are swollen and vacuolated. There are also areas of frank necrosis and inflammatory infiltration (H & E, 1,500×).

Other findings included internal hydrocephalus. There was focal necrosis and granuloma formation within the brain (Figs. 156 and 157), in the eye (Figs. 345 and 346), and in the adrenal (Fig. 317), all associated with *Toxoplasma* organisms.

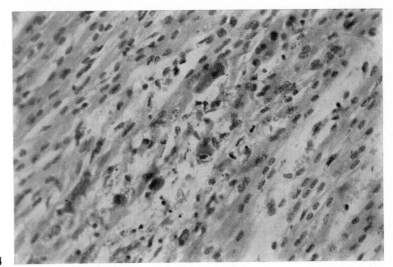

114

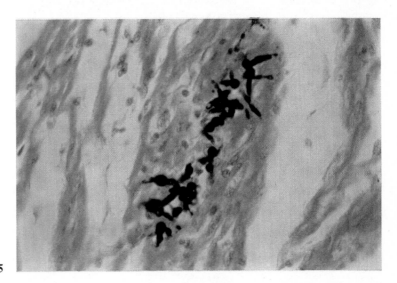

115

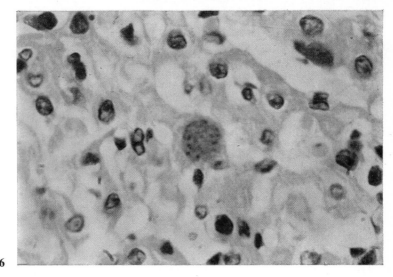

116

117
CONGENITAL CHAGAS' DISEASE

Male weighing 3,500 gm. Unknown gestational age. Admitted for splenomegaly and acute anemia. The mother was known to have typical Chagas' disease, confirmed by culture in an intermediate host. The infant died 24 hours after birth. (This case was seen by one of us in Brasilia, Brazil. Specimens from the autopsy were made available to us through the courtesy of Professor Marcio Lisboa, Medical Faculty of Brasilia.)

Histopathologic Examination. Within the myocardial tissue there is an accumulation of minute corpuscles in each of which the nucleus stands out because of its more intense basophilia. There is no inflammatory reaction (H & E, 1,500×).

Similar aggregates of parasites, identified as *Trypanosoma cruzi,* were observed in the placenta, lung, and liver.

118
CARDIAC GLYCOGENOSIS

Full-term male, weighing 3,000 gm, admitted on the fourth day of life because of refusal to nurse for 24 hours, dyspnea, expiratory whine, sclerema, and generalized hypotonia for 7 hours. At examination there were poor general condition, weak response to stimuli, pallor, perioral cyanosis, and 2 fingerbreadths' hepatomegaly. Chest films showed grade III cardiomegaly of global type. Pulmonary vasculature was concealed by cardiac enlargement. Radial and femoral pulses were palpable but weak. There were no murmurs. Three-tone rhythm identified by phonocardiography as representing atrial gallop. The phonocardiographic second sound was physiologically split with strong 2P. ECG showed sinus rhythm at 145 per minute.

All leads showed a remarkably diffuse disturbance of repolarization. In view of these findings a diagnosis of primary endomyocardopathy was considered or possibly hypoplasia of left chambers in one of the forms that may be associated with fibroelastosis. Digitalization was started. Blood sugar, 60 mg/100 ml, pH 7.10, pCO_2 55 mm Hg, BE -14.5 mEq/L. In spite of all therapeutic measures the infant died 24 hours later.

Histopathologic Examination. The heart was large, weighing 38 gm, as compared to a normal value of 19 gm. There was uniform thickening of cardiac walls without distortion of shape. Microscopically, the clear and vacuolated appearance of the fibers is striking; the myofibrillary substance is reduced to a peripheral ring (H & E, 600×).

PAS staining brought out a considerable accumulation of glycogen within myocardial fibers; there were no such deposits in other organs. Other findings: Massive pulmonary hemorrhage and severe fatty change limited to the right lobe of the liver.

119
CARDIOMEGALY IN OFFSPRING OF DIABETIC MOTHER

Female weighing 2,750 gm. Gestational age, 32 weeks. Apgar score 3 at birth, resuscitation required. It was the third pregnancy of this diabetic woman. Two previous conceptions had ended in abortion.

On admission the child's general condition was below par. The face and extremities were edematous, the liver was down 3 fingerbreadths; there were generalized cyanosis of moderate degree, hypotonia, and weakness of spontaneous movements. Chest radiographs suggested hyaline membrane disease. Mixed metabolic and respiratory acidosis. Blood sugar 30 mg/100 ml. Hypertonic dextrose and 1 M bicarbonate were administered. Eight hours after admission generalized myoclonic seizures appeared, as well as rapid, irregular respiration and intercostal retraction. The infant died 2 hours later.

Histopathologic Examination. The heart was enlarged, weighing 24 gm, but showed normal configuration. Microscopically, there is marked hypertrophy of the muscle fibers, which exhibit large nuclei of irregular sizes (H & E, 600×).

There was also pulmonary atelectasis accompanied by hyaline membranes. The pancreas exhibited hypertrophy and hyperplasia of the islets (Figs. 227 and 228). The kidney showed immaturity with persistence of the fetal zone.

Cardiac hypertrophy is a component of the visceromegalic syndrome seen in children of diabetic mothers. The heart and the liver are particularly affected, while the kidneys and the brain are often normal in weight. Extramedullary hematopoiesis is another frequent finding in these infants. The placenta may show endarteritis and thrombosis.

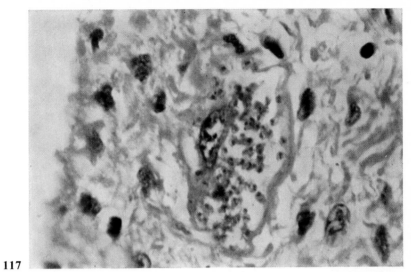

117

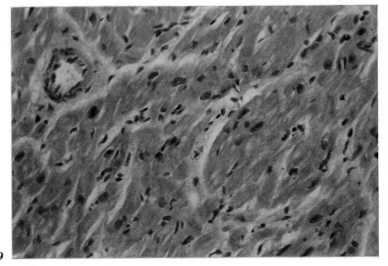

118

119

120
CARDIOMEGALY IN ERYTHROBLASTOSIS

Male weighing 2,210 gm. Gestational age, 35 weeks. Delivery by caesarean section. Apgar score 4 at birth. Blood group O, Rh (D) positive. Positive direct Coombs test. Hematocrit 30 per cent. Moribund on admission, with pale skin and mucosae, oozing umbilical cord, general hypotonia, and deficient respiration. Heart rate too rapid to be counted. An apneic crisis was successfully treated with intubation and assisted respiration. There was serious metabolic acidosis. Bicarbonate and dextrose solution were administered. Before exchange transfusion could be attempted, however, death ensued.

Histopathologic Examination. The heart weighed 40 gm. Considerable enlargement of myocardial nuclei can be seen microscopically, together with a certain degree of anisokaryosis. Within the interstitial capillaries there are erythroblasts (H & E, 600×).

Other findings: Active hematopoiesis especially in the liver and spleen; the septal capillaries of the lung contained abundant erythroblasts.

121
CONGENITAL FIBROSIS OF MYOCARDIUM. TRIPLOIDY

Male weighing 2,430 gm. Gestational age, 40 weeks. Delivered by cesarean section. Placenta with hydatidiform molar degeneration. History of jaundice in the mother in the tenth week of pregnancy. Admitted at 3 hours of life because of multiple malformations. Detailed history given with Figures 188 to 191 and 292 and 293. Karyotyping revealed triploidy with 69 chromosomes in a peripheral blood count. Death occurred at 36 hours.

Histopathologic Examination. The heart weighed 18 gm and showed no gross anomaly. The microscopic pattern was irregular, with rather large areas of fibrosis. Figure 121 demonstrates an irregular myocardial arrangement with disruption of the myocardial architecture created by loose connective tissue and marked histiocytic proliferation (H & E, 375×).

For other autopsy data, see Figures 188 to 191 and 292 and 293.

122
HEMORRHAGE INTO PAPILLARY MUSCLES

Female weighing 2,270 gm. Gestational age, 38 weeks. Forceps delivery in cephalic presentation. Meconium-tinged amniotic fluid. At birth, anoxia necessitated intubation, aspiration, and oxygen therapy. Borderline recovery. Admitted at 2 hours.

On admission, there were poor general condition, peripheral collapse, no spontaneous movements, brownish secretions in nose and mouth, as well as subcostal retraction, bradycardia, and no response to stimuli. Chest radiographs showed right-sided pulmonary emphysema and mediastinal shift. Vague micronodular shadows in the right upper lung field and the lower hilar area on the same side. pH 7.02, pCO_2 55 mm Hg, BE −17 mEq/L, microhematocrit 57 per cent.

Treatment with 1 M bicarbonate and dextrose, and incubator under standard conditions, without success. Death occurred 24 hours later.

Histopathologic Examination. In the center of Figure 122 there is a collection of blood surrounded by edematous myocardium undergoing necrosis. Myocardial fibers at some distance from the hemorrhagic area appear normal (H & E, 187.5×).

Other findings were aspiration pneumonia and intracerebral hemorrhagic foci.

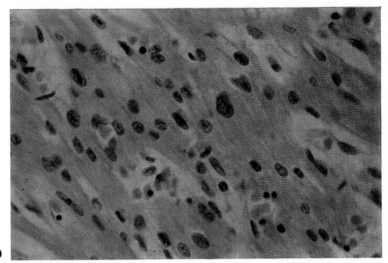

120

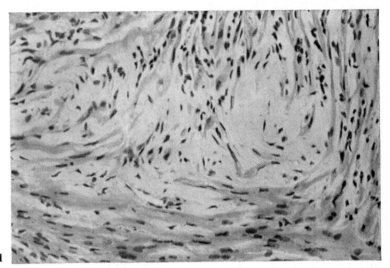

121

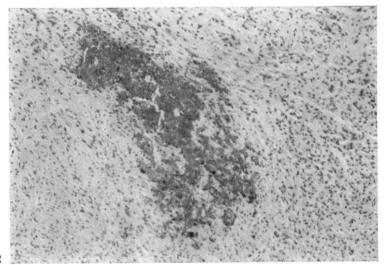

122

123
PERICARDIAL PETECHIAE CAUSED BY ANOXIA

Male weighing 1,500 gm. Gestational age, 28 weeks. Primiparous delivery after 22 hours' labor. Cephalic presentation. Apgar score 3 at birth.

Admitted at 6 hours, with marked hypotonia, generalized cyanosis, abnormal breathing, muffled heart sounds, and absence of basic reflexes. Despite assisted respiration and oxygen, death occurred 3 hours later.

Histopathologic Examination. Numerous petechiae were visible on the surface of the epicardium, especially in the vicinity of the coronary sinus and along the course of the coronary vessels.

Figure 123 shows a well-delimited hemorrhage within the epicardium, accompanied by capillary dilatation. It does not encroach on the myocardium (H & E, 187.5 ×).

There were also signs of serious anoxia manifested by the presence of petechiae, particularly conspicuous in the thymus, meninges, and pleural surfaces. The lungs showed congestive atelectasis with septal and perivascular hemorrhages and scanty evidence of hyaline membranes.

124
FOCAL FIBROSIS WITH CALCIFICATION

Female weighing 1,600 gm. Gestational age, 32 weeks. Admitted at 10 days because of diarrhea and dehydration. Mixed acidosis: pH 7.03, pCO_2 53 mm Hg, BE −19.5 mEq/L, microhematocrit 33 per cent. Stool culture yielded numerous colonies of *Candida albicans, Proteus,* and type O:111 B:4 *E. coli.*

After a temporary period of improvement following the use of fluids and antibiotics and treatment of acidosis, signs of gastroenteritis recurred, with sepsis and sustained acidosis. Death occurred 3 days later.

Histopathologic Examination. Figure 124 shows a small area of fibrosis in a papillary muscle, without inflammatory infiltration. The outlines of the area are not clear, especially toward the upper right corner. The presence of calcium deposits within the fibrous tissue is quite obvious (H & E, 375 ×). In the brain there were also small isolated calcific foci. They probably represent dystrophic calcification of damaged tissues.

Other findings: Necrotizing enteritis, bacterial pneumonia, and immaturity.

125
FIBROSIS OF PAPILLARY MUSCLES

Twenty-five day old male weighing 2,000 gm at birth. He remained in the hospital for 17 days and was discharged in apparently good condition. Eight days later he developed respiratory difficulty, restlessness, refusal to nurse, and vomiting of food, all without fever.

On admission his condition was poor; breathing and heart rate were rapid. Heart sounds were muffled. The membranes were dry, and there was metabolic acidosis.

Chest x-rays showed generalized pulmonary emphysema. Two hours after admission he died.

Histopathologic Examination. The heart weighed 20 gm. There were no gross changes.

Under the microscope many of the papillary muscles, especially those in the left ventricle, showed areas of central fibrosis such as is illustrated in Figure 125 (H & E, 125 ×). These areas were characterized by relatively acellular fibrous tissue replacing muscle fibers; inflammatory infiltration was not in evidence. These fibrotic foci were poorly outlined; slender fibrous tracts crept into myocardial muscle bundles.

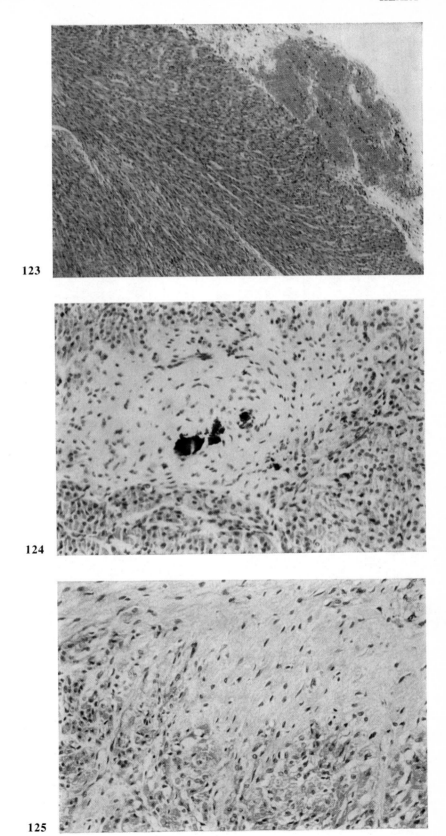

123

124

125

INFARCTION OF PAPILLARY MUSCLES

Male weighing 1,100 gm. Gestational age, 26 weeks. Apgar score 7 at birth. Admitted 1 hour after delivery showing obvious signs of immaturity, loss of muscle tone, and respiratory deficit. Placed in an incubator under standard conditions; the clinical course was fairly good for a week, but then respiratory difficulties recurred. Mixed acidosis was signaled by values of: pH 7.21, pCO_2 57 mm Hg, BE −6.5 mEq/L. The respiratory component became more serious, and death ensued on the following day.

Histopathologic Examination. Figure 126 shows a cross section of a papillary muscle with central foci of necrobiosis characterized by deeply eosinophilic staining and nuclear pyknosis. The borders of the lesions are poorly outlined. The vessels in the healthy portions of the myocardium are dilated and engorged (H & E, 187.5×). In other portions of the myocardium there were lesions similar to those depicted here, most of them close to the endocardial surface.

Other autopsy findings included marked visceral immaturity and severe congestive atelectasis.

EARLY MYOCARDIAL NECROSIS

Male infant weighing 1,080 gm; 32 weeks' gestational age. At 48 hours there was vomiting with abdominal distention, marked jaundice, pallor, and generally poor condition. On admission the infant appeared to be in acute respiratory failure and moribund. pH 6.83, pCO_2 90 mm Hg, BE −13.5 mEq/L. Chest x-ray showed pronounced reticulogranular pattern with a negative air bronchogram. Three hours after admission the infant died.

Histopathologic Examination. Figure 127 illustrates an irregular area of myocardium characterized by marked eosinophilia of the muscle fibers with homogenization of cytoplasm and loss of striations. The nuclei are pyknotic or karyorrhectic. There is neither hemorrhage nor inflammatory infiltration (H & E, 375×).

These foci of myocardial necrosis were numerous and predominant at the subendocardial level and in the papillary muscles. The coronary arteries were normal.

Autopsy also disclosed the presence of hemorrhagic pneumonia with numerous thrombi, passive congestion of the liver with necrotizing granulomas, subarachnoid hemorrhagic foci, and signs of immaturity including a continuous nephrogenic zone.

FIBROSIS OF MYOCARDIUM ACCOMPANIED BY RECENT NECROSIS

Two thousand eight hundred gram male. Gestational age, 40 weeks. Normal vertex delivery. At birth there were signs of anoxia requiring resuscitation. Admitted at 9 hours of life because of cyanosis, predominantly facial, shallow breathing with irregular rhythm, and marked loss of tone. Heart sounds were weak without murmur. The heart rate was slow, and there was 3 fingerbreadths' hepatomegaly.

Arterial pulses were palpable throughout. The second heart sound was physiologically split. Electrocardiogram at 10 hours showed pointed P wave in lead II and extreme right leads, as well as marked incomplete right bundle branch block. The tracing suggested right-sided enlargement, even considering the normal fetal pattern of right predominance. Chest x-ray showed grade 3 cardiomegaly. The heart rate was slow at 115 per minute.

A few hours later, left-sided tonic-clonic convulsions appeared. The total clinical picture became progressively worse. Bouts of apnea set in, and spontaneous movements ceased. pH 7.35, pCO_2 56 mm Hg, BE +2 mEq/L, microhematocrit 78 per cent. Despite digitalization and oxygen therapy, death supervened at 4 days of life.

Histopathologic Examination. The heart was moderately enlarged (30 gm) and presented no anomalies. Great vessels were normal. Microscopically there were many areas of necrobiosis, irregular in outline, as shown in Figure 128, with eosinophilic homogenization of fibers, most conspicuous in the walls of both ventricles and in the interventricular septum (H & E, 187.5×). In addition there were other, older lesions with fibrous replacement of the infarcted area.

Figure 129 shows an area of early fibrosis. Note the presence of muscle fiber remnants in the midst of this area (reddish fragments) and vacuolization of fibers at the junction with normal myocardium (Masson, 375×).

Other autopsy findings included foci of encephalomalacia, diapedesis of blood in kidneys and testicles, hemorrhagic bronchopneumonia, erosive esophagitis (Fig. 212) and early ischemic enteritis (Fig. 217).

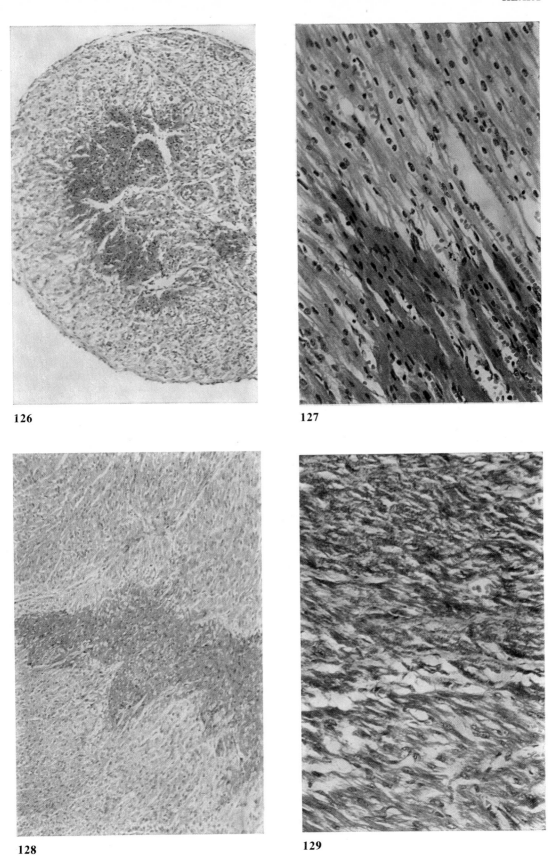

126

127

128

129

130/131
CALCIFICATION OF PULMONARY ARTERY

Male weighing 2,400 gm. Gestational age, 37 weeks. Normal cephalic delivery. During the third month of gestation the mother had an exanthem diagnosed as rubella.

The infant was admitted 3 hours after delivery in poor general condition, hypotonic, with generalized cyanosis, limited spontaneous movements, respiratory difficulty, and multiple malformations, including an ulcerated myelomeningocele, ulcerated omphalocele with herniation of the liver and intestines, microcephaly with a 28 cm cranial perimeter, hare lip with completely cleft palate, and polydactyly involving both hands and the right foot. Karyotype was normal. Death occurred 12 hours after admission.

Histopathologic Examination. Figure 130 shows focal destruction of the arterial wall accompanied by polymorphonuclear infiltration; linear, deeply basophilic streaky deposits stand out (H & E, 375×).

Figure 131 shows moderate thickening of the tunica interna. More conspicuous is the deposition of calcium salts, particularly adhering to the elastic fibers. The deposits are seen in the form of basophilic bands and, with von Kossa's calcium stain, as black-staining streaks (375×).

Other autopsy findings, apart from the already mentioned multiple malformations, were arhinencephaly and bilateral renal dysplasia.

132/133
RHABDOMYOMA OF THE HEART

Female weighing 2,500 gm. Gestational age, 29 weeks. Apgar score 5 at birth. Resuscitation had to be employed. Admitted 30 minutes later with cyanosis, intercostal retraction, hypotonia, and moderate edema of legs. The liver was palpable 3 fingerbreadths below the costal margin. Chest x-ray showed moderate mottling in the lower right lung field. pH 7.20, pCO_2 55 mm Hg, BE —7.8 mEq/L. At 6 hours of life she expelled small amounts of blood by mouth; this was repeated in the subsequent few hours. Jaundice appeared with 7.5 mg/100 ml total bilirubin. Heart sounds were clear at 130 per minute. Respiratory difficulty, however, increased, as did the hepatomegaly and edema. Death occurred at 48 hours.

Cultures of meconium, gastric contents, and cerebrospinal fluid were negative.

Histopathologic Examination. Heart: Figure 132 represents a section of the lateral wall of the left ventricle. Note a well-circumscribed nodule of light staining quality that protrudes into the lumen of the ventricle (H & E, 15×).

Figure 133 shows an area of the lesion at greater magnification; it demonstrates the type of voluminous muscle cells that make up the nodule. These cells have abundant, light-staining cytoplasm. Some of them show a "spider" arrangement of myofibrils around the nucleus (H & E, 175×). There were no hamartomatous lesions suggestive of tuberous sclerosis in other organs.

Autopsy revealed extensive hemorrhagic foci in both lungs, generalized visceral congestion, and petechiae in the brain, thymus, and myocardium.

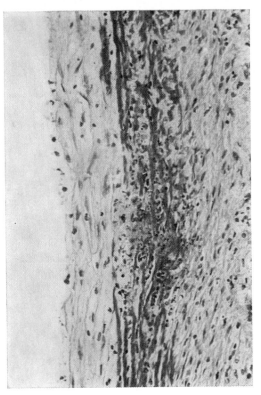

130

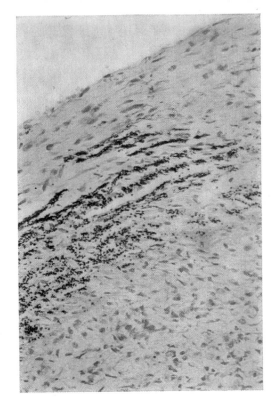

131

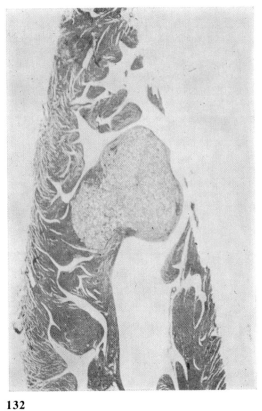

132

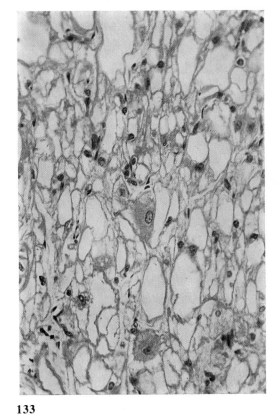

133

134
FUSIFORM ANEURYSM OF DUCTUS ARTERIOSUS WITH THROMBOSIS

Twenty-two day old female weighing 3,450 gm admitted for dehydration following a bout of acute gastroenteritis. Metabolic acidosis: pH 7.07, pCO_2 31 mm Hg, BE −21 mEq/L. Moribund condition. Bile-stained vomitus. Despite rehydration and treatment of acidosis, she died 6 hours later.

Histopathologic Examination. The ductus arteriosus showed fusiform aneurysmal dilatation. It was patent but exhibited mural thrombosis. The right-sided chambers were not hypoplastic. Figure 134 shows persistence of the internal elastica of the ductus, absence of the intima and presence of a relatively recent adherent thrombus. The fibrin network of the thrombus is stained brown (Verhoeff, 60×). In other areas there was organization of the thrombus.

Other autopsy findings: Acute bilateral pyelonephritis, left perinephric abscess, bilateral megaureter, and hypertrophic hemorrhagic cystitis.

135
ARTERITIS OF MYOCARDIAL VESSELS

Female weighing 2,550 gm. Gestational age, 36 weeks. Admitted at 14 hours of life because of poor general condition, acrocyanosis, hypertonicity, and irritability. Apgar score 2 at birth.

Spinal tap yielded a cloudy, purulent fluid that contained gram-positive organisms. Culture was positive for type IV *Listeria,* serologically identified. Metabolic acidosis: pH 7.18, pCO_2 30 mm Hg, BE −17 mEq/L. Treatment consisted of ampicillin and bicarbonate infusion. Death occurred 13 hours after admission.

Histopathologic Examination. Many of the myocardial vessels show fibrinoid necrosis of the wall effacing the normal architecture. In some of them there is also granulocytic infiltration of the wall and surrounding tissues and perivascular edema. No lesions of this type were observed in any other organ (H & E, 375×).

The principal finding at autopsy was *Listeria* meningitis (Fig. 158), but there were no granulomas in any other organs.

136/137
FIBROELASTOSIS

Nineteen day old male weighing 3,410 gm. Admitted in critical condition, apparently moribund, with generalized hypotonia, some cyanosis, acidotic fetor oris, tachycardia, depressed sensorium, no response to stimuli, 3-fingerbreadth hepatomegaly, and muffled heart sounds.

He had begun to vomit 4 days before admission, refused to nurse, and had dyspnea and fever. pH 7.09, pCO_2 58 mm Hg, BE −18 mEq/L. Chest plates showed cardiomegaly. Assisted respiration, oxygen, and bicarbonate perfusion were employed, but the infant died 6 hours after admission.

Histopathologic Examination. The endocardium of the left ventricle is greatly thickened by fibrous connective tissue, which stains green with Masson's trichrome. There is also some perivascular fibrosis within the myocardium but no inflammatory component (Fig. 136, 60×).

Elastica stain (Verhoeff) demonstrates hyperplasia of elastic fibers in the areas of fibrosis; these are most abundant in the vicinity of the heart muscle (Fig. 137, 600×).

Other autopsy findings: Pulmonary hemosiderosis, intraventricular hemorrhage, intracerebral hemorrhage, and extramedullary hematopoiesis in the liver, spleen, and lung.

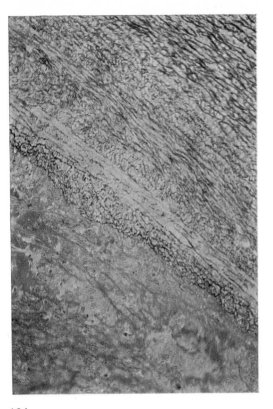

134

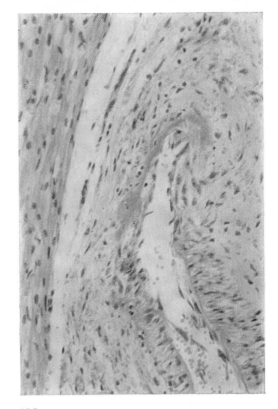

135

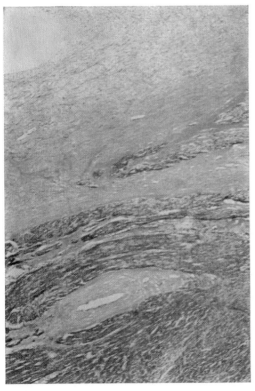

136

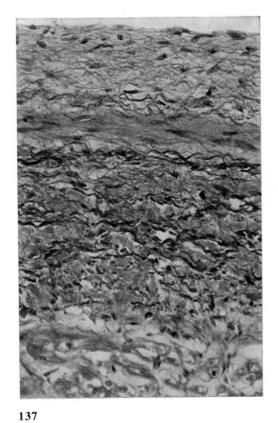

137

Central Nervous System

138
CEREBRAL IMMATURITY

Female weighing 540 gm. Gestational age, 25 weeks. Rupture of membranes 19 hours before delivery. Cephalic presentation. Apgar score 1 at birth, requiring energetic resuscitation. Admitted at 1 hour of life with generalized cyanosis, frank immaturity, weak heart sounds, bradycardia, and gasping respiration. pH 6.8, pCO_2 95 mm Hg, pO_2 breathing 100 per cent oxygen 50 mm Hg. No response to stimuli. Marked loss of tone. Attempt to correct acidosis by administering 1 M bicarbonate; assisted respiration, to no avail; death at 5 hours.

Histopathologic Examination. In the isocortex of the full-term infant layers number 1, 2, 3, and 4 can be readily distinguished, while 5 and 6 are much less apparent. Figure 138 shows this child's very immature brain, with considerable cellularity and no tendency to columnar transformation. The subpial zone is remarkably wide (H & E, 60×).

The autopsy also demonstrated rupture of a subcapsular hematoma of the liver leading to hemoperitoneum; petechiae in the thymus, lungs, and epicardium; bilateral intraventricular hemorrhage; and pulmonary anectasia.

139
CEREBELLAR IMMATURITY

Male weighing 1,230 gm. Gestational age, 32 weeks. Admitted 2 hours after delivery in poor general condition, with generalized cyanosis, moaning respiration, marked loss of tone, and overall immaturity. Chest films were suggestive of hyaline membrane disease. pH 7.12, pCO_2 88 mm Hg, blood sugar 120 mg/100 ml, arterial pO_2 in 100 per cent oxygen 60 mm Hg. Death occurred at 20 hours.

Histopathologic Examination. The molecular zone of the cerebellum still shows marked cellularity. There is a degree of disorganization of the Purkinje cells, and the granular zone sketches the formation of cerebellar "glomeruli" (H & E, 600×).

Other autopsy findings: Subarachnoid and brain stem hemorrhage, congestive pulmonary atelectasis with hyaline membranes, bilateral renal immaturity with wide continuous nephrogenic zone.

140
SUBCORTICAL CEREBELLAR HETEROTOPIC NIDUS

Female weighing 2,880 gm. Gestational age, 41 weeks. Admitted 15 hours after delivery. She appeared to be fairly well but had an expiratory whine and a weak cry. Examination showed acrocyanosis, low implantation of the ears, widened epicanthic folds, and cleft palate. Radiographic bone survey revealed only 11 pairs of ribs with hypoplasia of the superior ribs and fusion of the ossification centers of the sternum, duplication of some of the pedal phalanges, and an interorbital bony defect with malformation of the upper inner edge of the right orbit. Eye grounds were normal.

Cardiologic examination: Grade $^3/_6$ midsystolic murmur radiating to the back, thought to indicate a probable septal defect.

Karyotyping disclosed trisomy 13. At 17 days of age, she died with aspiration pneumonia.

Histopathologic Examination. Figure 140 shows a nidus of heterotopic, poorly organized tissue within the white substance of the cerebellum. It consists of large ganglion cells with eosinophilic cytoplasm mingling with streaks of cells reminiscent of the granular layer of the cerebellum (H & E, 375×). Other findings: Arrhinencephaly with agenesis of olfactory tracts, anomalies of osteogenesis, postsupracristal interventricular communication, cribriform foramen ovale, bicornuate uterus, agenesis of the gallbladder, accessory spleens, aberrant pancreatic tissue in the duodenum, and aspiration pneumonia.

141
ANENCEPHALY

Male weighing 3,400 gm. Gestational age, 44 weeks. Admitted 15 minutes after delivery in cardiorespiratory arrest, moribund. The infant was a typical anencephalic with generalized hypotonia who survived for 3 hours.

Histopathologic Examination. The brain was represented by an amorphous, friable mass, highly vascular and hemorrhagic, containing cystic cavities filled with clear fluid.

Figure 141 shows the microscopic architecture of the tissue. There are dilated vessels filled with erythrocytes and cavities with neuroepithelial lining. Glial tissue is also present (H & E, 375×).

The adrenals were very hypoplastic and lacked a fetal zone.

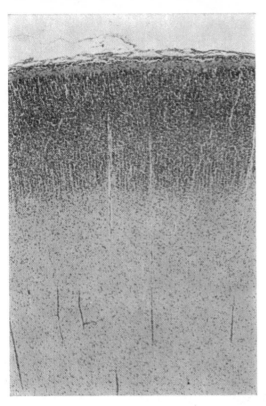

138

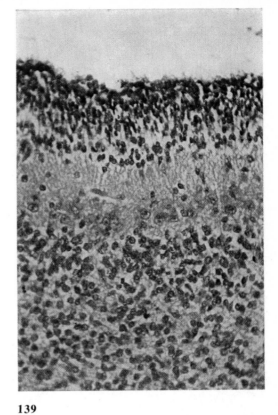

139

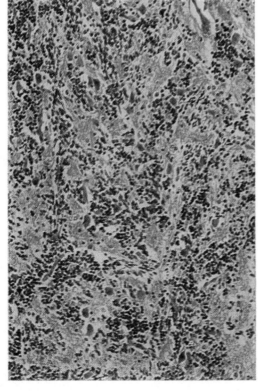

140

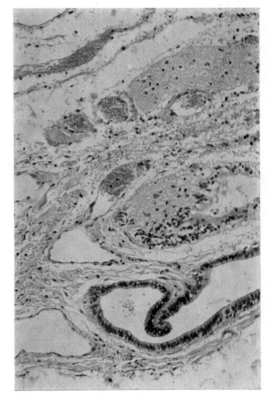

141

142
INTRAVENTRICULAR HEMORRHAGE

Female weighing 650 gm. Gestational age, 22 weeks. Rupture of membranes 4 days prior to delivery. Apgar score 1 at birth, requiring resuscitation. Admitted 30 minutes later, appearing generally quite immature, with gasping respirations, slow heart rate, areflexia, and generalized cyanosis. Chest films showed large unexpanded areas of the lungs. Death occurred 2 hours after birth.

Histopathologic Examination. On the right in Figure 142, the ependymal lining of the lateral ventricle is seen. Periventricular brain tissue shows marked cellularity, in keeping with the marked degree of immaturity of the child. On the left there is a greatly dilated vessel and a large area of hemorrhage (H & E, 187.5×). Grossly, the ventricular cavities were filled with blood. Other findings were: Diffuse congenital pneumonia, extensive atelectasis, and signs of immaturity in all organs.

143
SUBARACHNOID HEMORRHAGE

Female weighing 1,940 gm. Gestational age, 32 weeks. Admitted at 6 days of age in serious condition. For 2 days there had been loss of tone, whining, and perioral cyanosis. On admission she had hypothermia and hypotonia, generalized cyanosis, respiratory difficulty, altered sensorium, and pronounced intercostal retraction. Spinal fluid was hemorrhagic. Chest x-rays showed bilateral diffuse infiltration, more accentuated at the bases. Resuscitation and supportive treatment were administered. Two hours later hemoptysis and apnea supervened, and the infant died.

Histopathologic Examination. The subarachnoid space contains blood. Underlying brain is immature. Neurons are irregularly distributed without formation of layers (H & E, 187.5×). Other autopsy findings: Bronchopneumonia with areas of hemorrhage.

144
INTRACEREBELLAR HEMORRHAGE

Male weighing 3,300 gm. Gestational age, 38 weeks. Admitted at 48 hours. Apgar score 3 at birth. On admission he appeared very pale and in poor condition, with irregular breathing, intercostal retraction and expiratory whine, hypertonia, hyperreflexia, and hypothermia. The abdomen was distended. Spinal tap yielded cloudy, hemorrhagic fluid; culture was positive for *Listeria*, type IV. He died 24 hours after admission.

Histopathologic Examination. Figure 144 shows a number of hemorrhagic foci (diapedesis); the most prominent, at the center, is located in the granular layer of the cerebellum. Other foci can be seen in the molecular layer near the surface. Purkinje cells appear normal (H & E, 375×).

Other findings: Subarachnoid hemorrhage, focal intracerebral hemorrhages, and disseminated granulomatous listeriosis involving the liver, lymph nodes, adrenals, and lungs.

145
BRAIN STEM HEMORRHAGE

Male weighing 1,200 gm. Twin birth. Gestational age, 36 weeks. Admitted at 2 hours in serious condition with signs of dysmaturity, microcephaly, divergent strabismus, severe hypotonia, and pallor. Chest films showed a medium grade cardiomegaly. Cultures of blood, meconium, spinal fluid, and umbilical exudate were all negative. Gastric contents were positive for *Aerobacter aerogenes*. There was gradual general deterioration; respiratory arrest and death followed 36 hours after admission.

Histopathologic Examination. Grossly, the brain appeared normal. Microscopic study revealed the presence of small hemorrhagic foci within the basal ganglia and in the brain stem. Figure 145 shows such a lesion in the pons (H & E, 375×).

Aside from signs of immaturity, there were no other significant findings.

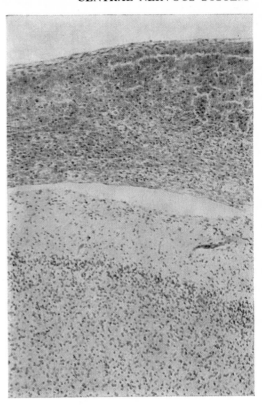

143

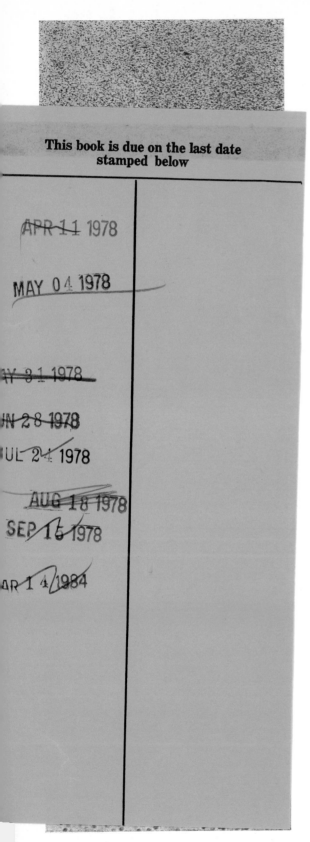

144

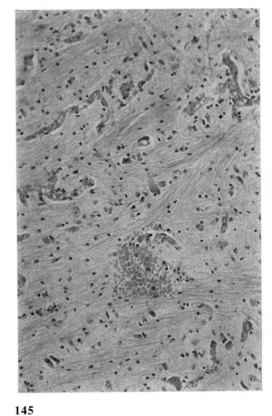

145

146
ENCEPHALOCELE

Female weighing 3,400 gm. Gestational age, 40 weeks. Admitted at 1 hour of life with microcephaly and a mass the size of a small orange projecting from the midoccipital region. The diagnosis of encephalocele was made. Surgery was performed 2 weeks later. The postoperative course was uneventful.

Histopathologic Examination. Tissue taken during the procedure is shown. In the superficial dermis there are hair follicles and sebaceous glands, shown here in cross section. Nearby, at a deeper level, there are bands of glial tissue (H & E, 60×).

Meningoceles, by contrast, do not show glial tissue.

147/148/149
GIANT CEREBRAL TERATOMA

Female weighing 2,480 gm. Gestational age, 33 weeks. Hydramnios. Admitted 15 minutes after birth in critical condition, with gasping respiration, extreme pallor, hydrocephalic appearance, marked hypotonia, and bradycardia. She died 15 minutes after admission. Cranial perimeter was 47 cm; thoracic 23. The skull had the consistency of parchment over some areas. There were paper-thin bones in the vault, and the sutures and fontanelles were greatly widened.

Histopathologic Examination. Cranial cavity contents: When the meninges were incised, an irregularly shaped, partially lobulated, partially cystic mass was exposed. It was friable and gelatinous, and showed no trace of cerebral cortical markings. Its total weight was 501 gm. Sections revealed cavities filled with yellowish fluid and multiple foci of calcification. The cerebellum had an immature appearance. The sella turcica and the orbital globes were normal. Microscopic examination demonstrated the presence of various types of mature tissues with predominance of neuroepithelial structures.

Figure 147 shows nervous tissue with a neuroepithelial tube (H & E, 375×).

Figure 148 shows, above, hyaline cartilage surrounded by a band of bone with two centers of ossification below (Masson, 375×).

Figure 149 illustrates the presence of striated muscle (Masson, 600×).

Other types of tissue encountered were squamous epithelium and glandular spaces lined by various kinds of epithelium.

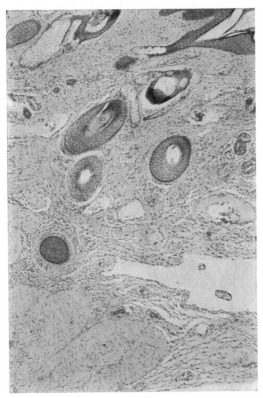

146

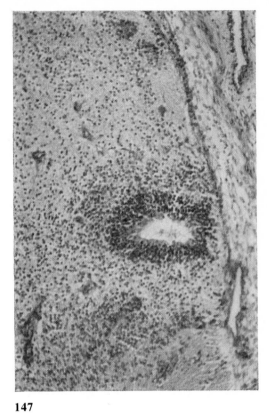

147

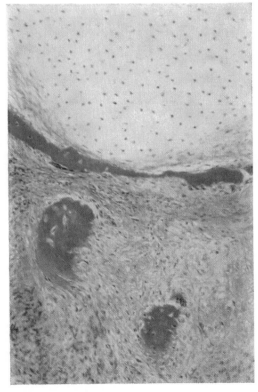

148

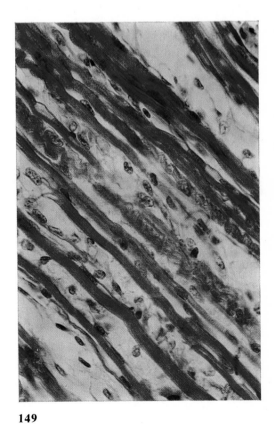

149

150/151
HEMORRHAGIC CUFFING ASSOCIATED WITH HYALINE CAPILLARY THROMBI

Female weighing 3,750 gm. Gestational age, 42 weeks. Cephalic delivery after 13 hours of labor. Apgar score 1 at birth, necessitating brisk resuscitation with intubation and assisted respiration. On admission, 1 hour after birth, her condition was very serious. There was no response to stimuli, muscle tone was very deficient, and reflexes were absent. Assisted respiration had to be maintained. Chest radiographs suggested a diagnosis of aspiration pneumonia. pH 7.21, pCO_2 44 mm Hg, BE −11 mEq/L, microhematocrit 63 per cent. Bicarbonate 1 M solution and 10 per cent dextrose were administered intravenously. Improvement was observed, and assisted respiration was discontinued at 24 hours of life. Twelve hours later, however, a new apneic crisis occurred, her general condition worsened, and she died despite efforts at resuscitation.

Histopathologic Examination. Figure 150 shows two perivascular cuffs of hemorrhagic infiltration. The erythrocytes are stained blue by phosphotungstic acid–hematoxylin (375×).

With high magnification, fibrin thrombi are seen as a network of fibers oriented parallel to the direction of blood flow, an indication of coagulation in vivo (Fig. 151, PTA-H, 600×).

Other autopsy findings: Similar capillary thrombi in the glomeruli, right renal hemorrhagic infarct, and hemorrhagic bronchopneumonia.

152
ENCEPHALOMALACIA

Male weighing 3,500 gm. Gestational age, 42 weeks. Labor lasted 12 hours, culminating in a difficult and traumatic breech delivery. Two hours later the infant was admitted in respiratory arrest, moribund, with weak and slow heart beat, pallor, no spontaneous movements, hypotonia, and no reaction to stimuli. In the cervical region there was a circular ecchymosis. There was no response to resuscitative measures.

Histopathologic Examination. Figure 152 shows an area of encephalomalacia beginning to undergo cavitation. It contains scavenger cells that have engulfed lipid granules. Many neurons exhibit pyknotic, contracted nuclei that tend to take up peripheral positions (H & E, 375×).

Other autopsy findings were traumatic rupture of the clavicular bundle of the left sternocleidomastoid muscle and generalized signs of anoxia.

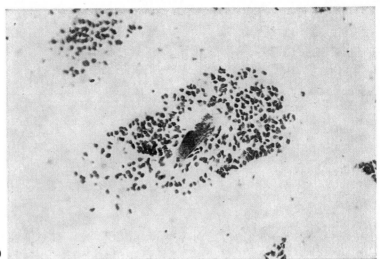

150

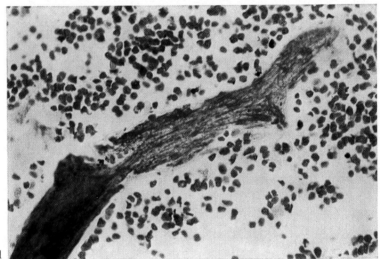

151

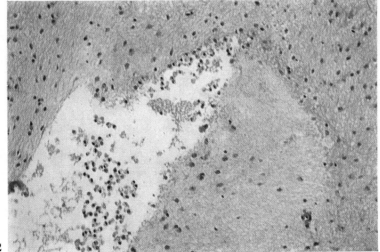

152

153
CEREBRAL CALCIFICATION

Male weighing 1,350 gm. Unknown gestational age. Admitted 1 hour after birth in poor condition. The face was abnormal; the ears were implanted below the normal site and were deformed. The anus was imperforate; the feet were clubbed; there were bilateral cataracts and unilateral cryptorchidism. Further investigation revealed the presence of esophageal atresia and tracheoesophageal fistula. Agenesis of kidneys and their excretory pathways was suspected. Death occurred 40 hours after admission.

Histopathologic Examination. The configuration of the brain was normal, and the weight correlated with that of the child. There was diffuse subarachnoid and also intraventricular hemorrhage. Microscopically, irregular foci of calcification were found. There was no inflammatory reaction, nor were there cytomegalic inclusions or any *Toxoplasma* granulomas (H & E, 187.5×).

Other autopsy findings: Annular pancreas, rectal atresia, bilateral agenesis of kidneys and urinary excretory tracts.

154/155
CYTOMEGALIC INCLUSION ENCEPHALITIS

Male weighing 2,800 gm. Gestational age, 38 weeks. Cephalic delivery with fetid, brownish amniotic fluid. Apgar score 7 at birth. Admitted at 3 hours of life in poor condition with few spontaneous movements but good response to stimuli, deep jaundice, diffuse purpura in skin and mucosa, and marked hepatosplenomegaly. Isoimmunization was ruled out by pertinent studies. Twenty-four hours later serum bilirubin was 20 mg/100 ml. Exchange transfusion was performed. Blood count showed 15,000 leukocytes per cubic millimeter and 30 per cent erythroblasts. Bone marrow study ruled out congenital leukemia. Chest films were normal. Spinal tap yielded slightly hemorrhagic fluid. Cultures of blood, urine, meconium, and spinal fluid were negative. The fundus of the right eye was normal; in the left eye there was a papillary hemorrhage. In succeeding hours myoclonus appeared in the extremities and the purpura worsened. Three examinations of the urine for cells with cytomegalic inclusions were negative. The infant died 40 hours after admission.

Histopathologic Examination. Figure 154 shows inflammatory foci consisting of round cells, with moderate glial proliferation. Cells with cytomegalic inclusions are evident. (H & E, 375×).

Other fields showed calcification, particularly around small blood vessels (Fig. 155, H & E, 187.5×).

Other findings: Cytomegalic cells in the lungs, liver, spleen, kidney, and thymus; subarachnoid hemorrhage and minimal intracerebral hemorrhage.

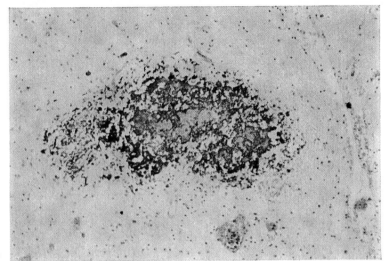

153

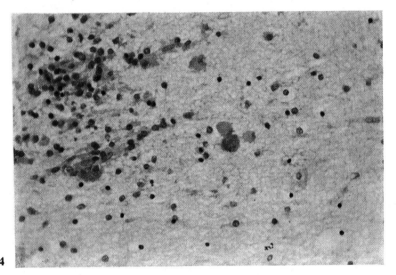

154

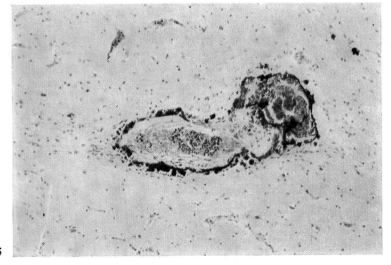

155

CONGENITAL TOXOPLASMOSIS

Female weighing 2,480 gm. Gestational age, 32 weeks. Case history is given with Figure 116. *Toxoplasma* immunofluorescence titer in mother and infant: 1:1,200.

Histopathologic Examination. Grossly, the cerebral cortex was thin and the ventricles were markedly dilated. There were extensive areas of calcification on the cortical surface. Figure 156 represents granulation tissue with distended vessels, marked round cell infiltration, and, below, irregular calcific deposits (H & E, 187.5×). Within the granulomas there are *Toxoplasma* cysts, two of them shown in Figure 157 (H & E, 1,500×).

In addition to microphthalmia the autopsy showed granulomas and *Toxoplasma* cysts in the globe of the eye (Figs. 356 and 357), adrenals (Fig. 317), and myocardium (Fig. 116).

LISTERIA MENINGITIS

Female weighing 2,250 gm; 36 weeks' gestational age. Apgar score 2 at birth, necessitating resuscitation. Case history is given with Figure 135. Admitted at 14 hours of age with generalized cyanosis and rapid breathing. The mother had suffered a febrile episode 10 days before delivery. She was a known diabetic and had an abundant vaginal discharge. On admission the infant was in fair condition, showing acrocyanosis, rapid breathing, hypertonicity, hypermotility, and a depressed fontanelle. The chest x-ray demonstrated scattered bilateral micronodular densities compatible with the diagnosis of listeriosis. Two hours after admission there were obvious right-sided convulsions including the facial musculature.

Spinal tap yielded cloudy fluid from which type IV *Listeria* was cultured. In spite of intensive treatment the infant died 13 hours after admission.

Histopathologic Examination. The subarachnoid space was widened, and the membrane was seeded with granulomas such as the one shown in Figure 158, ringing a capillary and consisting of mononuclear and polymorphonuclear cells (H & E, 375×).

Similar granulomas with a tendency toward necrosis were seen in both adrenals. Warthin-Starky stains revealed argyrophilic pleomorphic organisms that were also gram-positive.

There were also marked hyperplasia of the islets of Langerhans and arteritis of myocardial vessels (Fig. 135).

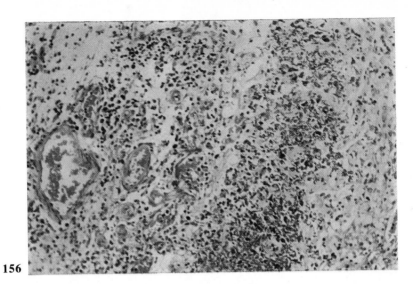

156

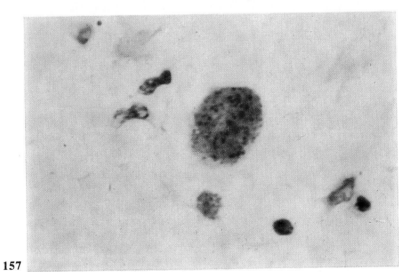

157

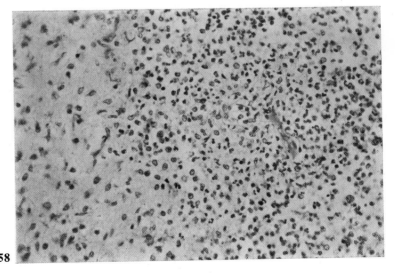

158

159
PURULENT LISTERIA CHOROIDITIS

Male infant weighing 1,200 gm. Gestational age, 29 weeks. Apgar score 4 at birth. Admitted at 30 minutes of life in very poor general condition, obviously immature, with respiratory difficulty, hypotonia, and diminished reflexes. Excessive mucus in the oropharynx. Chest x-ray showed confluent bilateral nodular densities. Pharyngeal exudate was positive for type IV *Listeria,* also demonstrable in gastric contents. After repeated apneic crises, the infant died at 30 hours of age. Meconium culture was negative.

Histopathologic Examination. The ependymal lining shows patches of denudation. The subependymal layer is markedly infiltrated by polymorphonuclear leukocytes. The choroid plexuses and the subarachnoid space exhibited similar infiltration (H & E, 60×).

Typical *Listeria* granulomas with organisms demonstrable by appropriate staining were seen in the adrenals, myocardium, and lungs.

160
E. COLI MENINGITIS

Male weighing 2,600 gm. Unknown gestational age. Admitted at age of 5 days, with jaundice and convulsions. He was in poor general condition, with intercostal retraction, deep jaundice, hyperactive reflexes, and generalized tonic-clonic convulsions. Bilirubin was 14.5 mg/100 ml. Tests for isoimmunization were negative. Spinal tap yielded purulent fluid; culture showed abundant colonies of *E. coli.* There was no response to intensive treatment, and convulsions recurred. Death occurred 7 days after admission.

Histopathologic Examination. On opening the skull a purulent meningeal collection was observed, chiefly on the surface of the right occipital lobe. The ventricles were filled with creamy pus that was positive for *E. coli.* Figure 160 shows subarachnoid thickening and infiltration by mononuclear cells with few neutrophils (H & E, 187.5×).

The remainder of the autopsy was noncontributory.

161
CANDIDA ALBICANS MENINGOENCEPHALITIS

Male weighing 2,950 gm. Unknown gestational age. Admitted at 6 days of life in poor general condition, with pronounced sclerema in the hands and feet, myoclonia in the upper extremities, and respiratory distress. The liver was enlarged, and there was an abdominal mass the size of a tangerine, smooth and movable, located anteriorly, and not in contact with the lumbar spine. Spinal fluid was somewhat cloudy but bacteriologically negative. Chest x-ray was compatible with aspiration pneumonia. Persistent metabolic acidosis was treated with bicarbonate infusion. Two days after admission the abdomen felt doughy, but the plain film showed no air-fluid levels nor any abnormal distribution of abdominal air shadows. Persistent myoclonias appeared in the eyelids and extremities, and there was marked hypertonicity generally.

Dorsal hemivertebrae were demonstrated. The infant's condition worsened; myoclonic seizures increased, and respiratory insufficiency appeared. At 13 days of life, the child died in a hemorrhagic crisis with expulsion of blood-tinged mucus.

Histopathologic Examination. Purulent exudate was found within the cerebral sulci. Microscopically, in addition to suppurative meningitis, there were numerous granulomas containing hyphae of *Candida albicans* within the cerebral parenchyma and also foci of encephalomalacia (Gomori, 375×).

Other findings: Enteric duplication cyst and aspiration pneumonia with a hemorrhagic component.

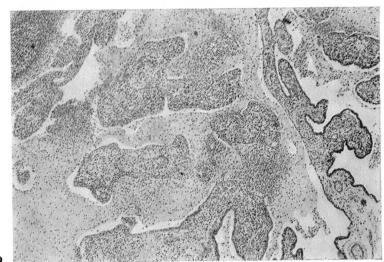

159

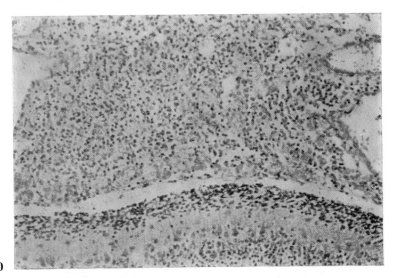

160

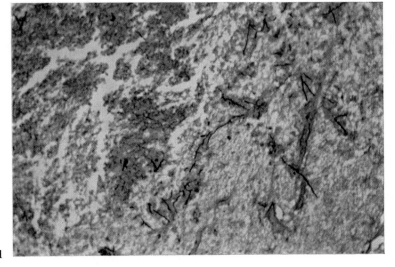

161

Kidney

162
RENAL IMMATURITY. NEPHROGENIC ZONE MARKED

Male weighing 640 gm. Gestational age, 22 weeks. Apgar score 3 at birth, necessitating energetic resuscitation. Admitted at 2 hours of life in poor general condition, with bouts of cyanosis and apnea. The course continued downhill despite all measures, and death occurred at 6 hours.

Histopathologic Examination. Grossly, the surface of the kidney showed lobulation. Figure 162 shows, under the capsule, a broad continuous nephrogenic zone. It includes rudimentary glomeruli. The distal segments of the nephrons show ampullary dilatation and invagination (H & E, 60×).

The remainder of the organs exhibited obvious signs of immaturity. The lungs were poorly expanded; there was peribronchial (iatrogenic) emphysema. A subcapsular hematoma of the liver was present. Petechiae were scattered abundantly over visceral surfaces.

163
RENAL IMMATURITY. NEPHROGENIC ZONE MODERATE

Male weighing 2,000 gm. Gestational age, 34 weeks. Admitted at 3 hours in poor general condition, with cyanosis and respiratory difficulty. Chest films showed typical hyaline membrane disease. pH 6.94, pCO_2 over 100 mm Hg, BE −33 mEq/L. Death at 10 hours, in respiratory arrest.

Histopathologic Examination. The nephrogenic zone is not as broad as in the preceding case. It is not continuous. The subcapsular glomeruli are well differentiated, as may be seen in Figure 163 (H & E, 187.5×).

Other findings: Subarachnoid hemorrhage and congestive pulmonary atelectasis with hyaline membranes.

164
RENAL IMMATURITY. NEPHROGENIC ZONE MINIMAL

Female weighing 2,800 gm. Gestational age, 39 weeks. Meconium-tinged amniotic fluid. Admitted 2 days after delivery with hyperthermia, respiratory difficulty, and refusal to nurse. On examination: Poor general condition, septic picture, generalized hypotonia, convergent strabismus, and bulging fontanelle. Spinal tap produced cloudy fluid from which pneumococci were isolated. Died of meningitis within 24 hours.

Histopathologic Examination. A few islands of nephrogenic tissue persist in the subcapsular zone, alternating with extensive areas of good glomerular differentiation. There are immature basophilic tubules in the superficial portions of the cortex (H & E, 60×).

Other autopsy findings: Massive amniotic fluid aspiration, bronchopneumonia, and suppurative meningitis.

165
RENAL IMMATURITY. REMNANTS OF NEPHROGENIC ZONE

Female weighing 3,200 gm. Unknown gestational age. Admitted at 4 hours because of poor general condition, cyanosis and respiratory distress, myelomeningocele, and anal atresia. Chest x-rays were suggestive of pulmonary hyaline membrane disease. She died 24 hours after admission.

Histopathologic Examination. The kidneys were grossly normal in shape, the weight proportionate to body weight. Microscopically, there was no nephrogenic zone as such, although here and there within the subcapsular area an occasional cluster of intensely basophilic tubules can be seen. The glomeruli show a degree of maturity commensurate with the age and weight of the child (H & E, 187.5×).

Other findings: Myelomeningocele, anal atresia, intestinal malrotation, vesicocolic fistula, and pulmonary hyaline membranes.

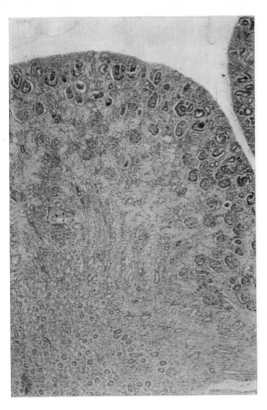

162

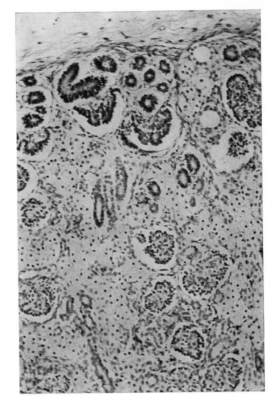

163

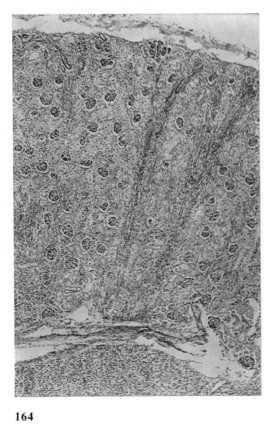

164

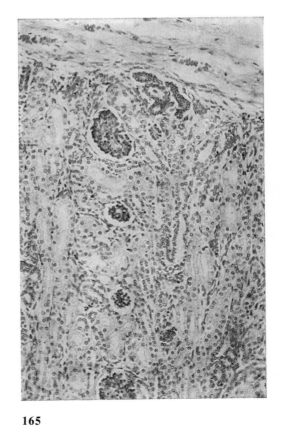

165

CONGENITAL GLOMERULOSCLEROSIS

Male weighing 3,650 gm. Gestational age, 40 weeks. Admitted at 7 days of life because of hypertonic seizures. Delivery had been by cesarean section. Apgar score 7 at birth. On examination, poor general condition, shallow breathing, hypertonicity, generalized hyperreflexia, bulging fontanelle, and opisthotonus were found. Spinal tap yielded hemorrhagic fluid. EEG revealed high-voltage spikes, predominantly anteriorly and at the vertex. Metabolic acidosis.

A diagnosis of cerebral hemorrhage was made. During subsequent days there were generalized convulsive seizures. Death occurred 4 days after admission.

Histopathologic Examination. Figure 166 shows a glomerulus in which there is almost complete hyalinization of the loop. Its surface is covered by epithelial cells corresponding to the lining of Bowman's capsule, with which they are continuous. Note the absence of any glomerular lumen (Masson, 600×).

Autopsy confirmed the presence of extensive intracerebral hemorrhages.

PARTIAL CONGENITAL GLOMERULOSCLEROSIS

Male weighing 2,400 gm. Gestational age, 37 weeks. Twin pregnancy in transverse presentation requiring version and extraction. Apgar score 0 at birth, requiring resuscitation with intubation and assisted respiration. Admitted at 7 hours of life in serious condition, with shallow respirations, marked depression, and hypotonia. Metabolic acidosis. A 1 M bicarbonate and 10 per cent dextrose solution was administered. Spinal tap produced hemorrhagic fluid. The next day repeated convulsions occurred. Bouts of apnea necessitated repeated intubation and assisted respiration. Death occurred on the third day of life.

Histopathologic Examination. The glomerulus shown in Figure 167 exhibits transformation of the right side of the loop into a hyaline mass partially covered by flattened epithelial cells. The rest of the glomerulus is normal for this age and weight (Masson, 600×).

Other findings: Massive subarachnoid hemorrhage and focal pulmonary hemorrhages.

FIBROSIS OF GLOMERULAR CAPSULE

Female weighing 3,250 gm. Gestational age, 39 weeks. Rupture of membranes 3 days prior to delivery. Apgar score 4 at birth. Admitted 30 minutes after delivery in poor general condition with respiratory distress, tachycardia, heart sounds displaced to the right, generalized cyanosis, and marked hypotonia. Chest films confirmed the tentative diagnosis of diaphragmatic hernia. Serious respiratory acidosis: pH 6.75, pCO_2 over 100 mm Hg, BE −21 mEq/L. After supportive measures, surgery was undertaken. A total left diaphragmatic hernia was encountered; contained in the left hemithorax were the left lobe of the liver, the stomach and intestinal tract down to the colon, the spleen, and the pancreas. Bilateral pulmonary hypoplasia could not be corrected. Death occurred on the operating table.

Histopathologic Examination. Figure 168 shows a glomerulus with some tumefaction of its cells. There is conspicuous concentric fibrosis of the capsule, especially noted when compared with two adjacent normal glomeruli (Masson, 375×).

Autopsy confirmed the presence of the aforementioned diaphragmatic hernia and pulmonary hypoplasia affecting principally the left lung.

CONGENITAL GLOMERULAR CYSTS

Female weighing 3,050 gm. Gestational age, 38 weeks, Greenish amniotic fluid. Apgar score 1 at birth. Energetic resuscitation was carried out, with restoration of rather shallow spontaneous respiration. Admitted at 1 hour of life with considerable respiratory deficit, hypotonia, areflexia, and marked bradycardia. Chest x-rays showed infiltrative lesions, especially in the right lung field, which were considered highly suggestive of aspiration pneumonia. Metabolic acidosis: pH 6.92 and BE −20 mEq/L. The infant died 10 hours after admission.

Histopathologic Examination. Figure 169 shows two renal corpuscles with some contraction of the glomerular tuft, more marked in the lower one. Cystic dilatation of the space of Bowman, occupied by serous fluid, is apparent (Masson, 375×).

Other findings: Generalized signs of anoxia and massive pulmonary aspiration.

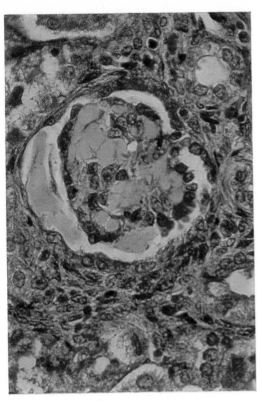

166

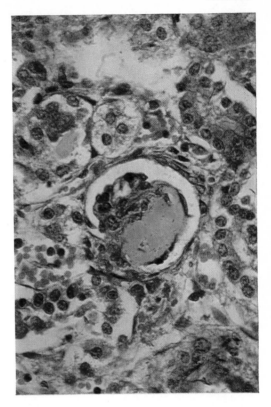

167

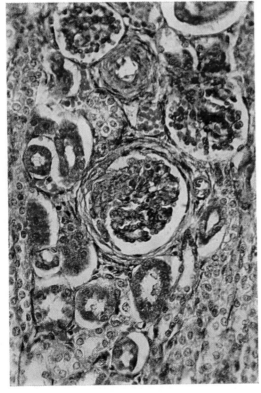

168

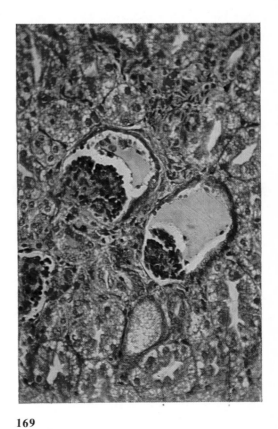

169

170
NODULE OF UNDIFFERENTIATED RENAL BLASTEMA

Female weighing 2,240 gm. Gestational age, 32 weeks. Normal delivery. Admitted at 3 hours of life. Physical features were characteristic of Down's syndrome. Twenty-four hours later intestinal obstruction developed. Roentgen films revealed a pattern of air-fluid levels to left and right of the epigastric region and absence of air shadows in the rest of the abdomen. The clinical impression was duodenal atresia. Laparotomy demonstrated an annular pancreas. Death supervened 36 hours after surgery.

Histopathologic Examination. In the subcapsular zone of the kidney there were several nests of cells with large nuclei containing loose chromatin and with scanty cytoplasm. One of these nests is shown in Figure 170. The sharp demarcation between the cell nest and the adjacent renal parenchyma is emphasized by the presence of a delicate connective tissue capsule surrounding the former. The peripheral cells of the nodule are arranged in a palisade, lining the inner aspect of the capsule. There is no capillary penetration nor any nephrogenic differentiation (H & E, 375×). The rest of the kidney was normal.

These nests of undifferentiated renal blastema appear with a frequency of 0.36 per cent in our series. Sixty-four per cent of them are associated with other types of malformation. They generally appear in the subcapsular zone, but may also appear deeper in the parenchyma, in connection with or unrelated to capsular sulci. They may be single or multiple, uni- or bilateral. Their significance is a matter of debate; some feel that they represent in situ Wilms' tumors. They are probably embryonal remnants with no growth tendency.

Autopsy also revealed annular pancreas and hemorrhagic broncopneumonia.

171
METAPLASTIC OSSIFICATION OF GLOMERULUS

Male weighing 3,400 gm. Gestational age, 38 weeks. Apgar score 10 at birth. Admitted at 24 hours of age because of weak cry and shallow breathing. On admission he was practically moribund, with gasping respirations, generalized cyanosis, marked hypotonia and areflexia, hypothermia, bulging fontanelle, bradycardia, and no corneal reflex. Resuscitation was successful. Metabolic acidosis: pH 7.02, pCO_2 46

mm Hg, BE —22 mEq/L. Spinal tap yielded hemorrhagic fluid. He was treated for acidosis. Bouts of apnea recurred, and death occurred 24 hours after admission.

Histopathologic Examination. Figure 171 shows a glomerulus with an ample capsular space partly occupied by a normal capillary tuft. The upper portion is occupied by an osseous plaque with well-defined lines of apposition and visible osteocytes. At the edge of this plaque there are cells that are reminiscent of osteoblasts found in normal bone. Note the presence of fat cells between the two components within the glomerular space (Masson, 375×). The lesion was solitary, and there were no changes in the rest of the parenchyma.

Other findings: Subdural and subtentorial intracranial hemorrhages, necrotizing tracheitis, and macrophages in alveoli.

172/173
OLIGOMEGANEPHRONIE

Male weighing 3,200 gm. Gestational age, 42 weeks. Apgar score 5 at birth. Admitted 1 hour later. Physical findings: Down's syndrome, intense cyanosis, poor general condition, respiratory insufficiency. Chest x-rays showed cardiomegaly. Cardiologic studies demonstrated a large interventricular septal defect. Evacuation of meconium was delayed; abdominal films showed distention of intestinal loops and direct visualization of meconium. Subsequent course was stormy. Weight was static. Diarrhea appeared on day 15. Two days later, he died.

Histopathologic Examination. The kidneys were small. The right weighed 4 gm and the left 8 gm. Outwardly they were not remarkable, except for size. Microscopically, in contrast to simple renal hypoplasia, the number of glomeruli was decreased and their size was increased (Fig. 172, H & E, 375×). This can be appreciated better by comparing this illustration with another (normal) kidney of an infant of the same age and weight (Fig. 173, H & E, 375×). The tubules are dilated, and the tubular epithelium is flattened. Most striking is the dilatation of the distal convoluted tubule with a very conspicuous macula densa that abuts against the glomerulus in Figure 172. The entire juxtaglomerular apparatus was quite prominent.

Other findings: A large interventricular septal defect was found. There was also acute necrotizing enteritis and fatty degeneration of the liver.

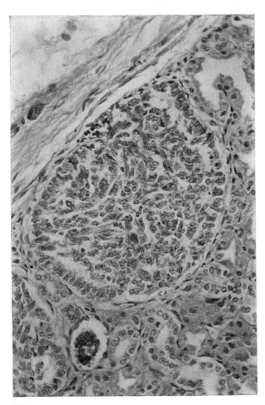

170

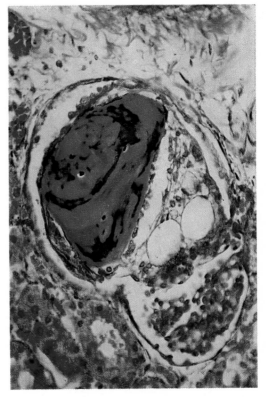

171

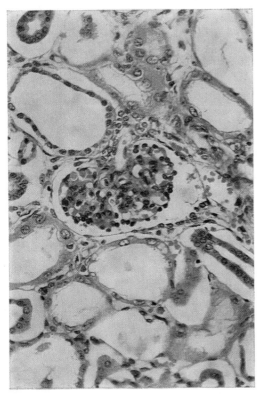

172

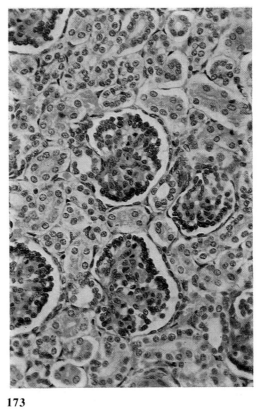

173

174/175
UNILATERAL HYPOPLASTIC-DYSPLASTIC KIDNEY

Male weighing 1,240 gm. Gestational age, 26 weeks. Apgar score 1 at birth. Admitted at 20 minutes of life, in poor general condition, breathing poorly, with generalized cyanosis, hypotonia, and edema of the legs. pH 7.04, pCO_2 78 mm Hg, BE -13 mEq/L. Chest x-rays were suggestive of hyaline membrane disease. Ten hours after admission the child died.

Histopathologic Examination. Grossly, the right kidney was normal; the left was small and irregular in shape, and showed multiple small cysts.

Figure 174 shows cysts of variable size replacing the normal architecture. The cysts are lined by flattened epithelium. The stroma is made up of fibrous tissue, with loose areas within which there are tubular structures of embryonal type (Masson, 60×).

Figure 175 shows the latter, embryonal areas with undifferentiated tubules lined by tall cylindrical epithelium, with large, chromatin-rich nuclei and spaces lined by pseudostratified epithelium (H & E, 600×).

Other findings: Congestive pulmonary atelectasis and pulmonary hyaline membrane disease.

176/177
BILATERAL DYSPLASTIC RENAL HYPOPLASIA

Male weighing 2,380 gm. Gestational age, 40 weeks. Cesarean delivery. Apgar score 2 at birth. Intensive resuscitation. Admitted at 2 hours of life, moribund, with respiratory distress, generalized hypotonia, cyanosis, weak heart sounds, and bradycardia. Facies was reminiscent of the Potter type. Chest x-ray suggested virtually total lack of expansion of the lungs. Death supervened 30 minutes after admission.

Histopathologic Examination. Both kidneys together weighed 10 gm. They were reduced to two nondescript cystic lumps with rudimentary ureters. Microscopically, the changes in the renal architecture were striking. Figure 176 shows an extensive area of fibrosis, a patch of stratified squamous epithelium, and an epidermal cyst containing a large keratin aggregate (Masson, 187.5×).

Figure 177 features a plaque of hyaline cartilage, embryonal tubular formations, and, below, two isolated glomeruli surrounded by dense connective tissue (Masson, 187.5×).

Other findings: Bilateral pulmonary anectasia and hypoplasia.

Comment: Reviewing 3,450 pediatric autopsies performed in this hospital we encountered 4 cases of unilateral renal dysplasia, 24 cases of bilateral renal dysplasia, and 7 cases of focal dysplasia. Malformations in other organs ranged from 5 per cent in the cases of unilateral dysplasia to 42.86 per cent in the cases of focal dysplasia and 91.47 per cent in the cases of bilateral dysplasia. There were no sex differences in the occurrence of both types of lesion. Unilateral hypoplasia-dysplasia is, nevertheless, the most frequently encountered disturbance of differentiation in the kidney. The actual number of cases reflected in our autopsy series indicates only that these infants survive if the malformations in other organs are not important.

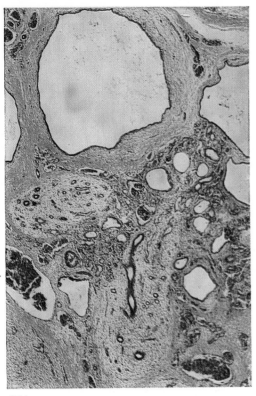

174

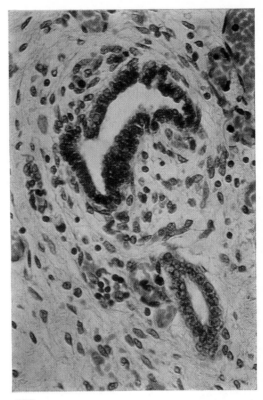

175

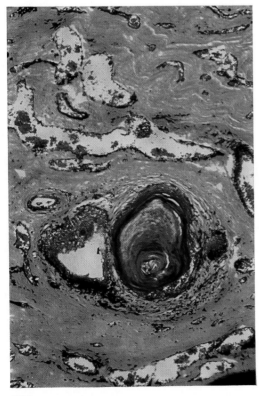

176

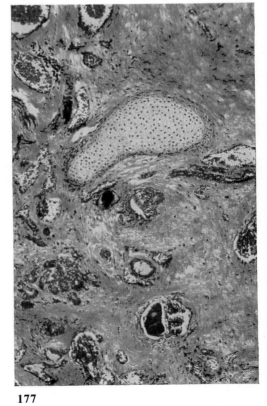

177

178
SEGMENTAL DYSPLASIA

Female weighing 4,100 gm. Gestational age, 44 weeks. Admitted at 20 days of life because of abdominal enlargement present from birth. On admission the infant appeared very pale and generally ill. The abdomen was enlarged and very tense. There was a prominent venous network. Palpation revealed a mass in the right infraumbilical region that was not clearly outlined but appeared to be related to the bladder. Abdominal films showed dilated intestinal loops displaced upward. Blood urea 91 mg/100 ml. Catheterization of the bladder reduced the volume of the mass. The diagnosis of congenital bilateral hydronephrosis was made. Death occurred on the day following admission.

Histopathologic Examination. Grossly, there was bilateral hydropyonephrosis and bilateral dolichomegaureter. The left kidney showed a microcystic nodule in the upper pole. This mass was partly necrotic. From it a third ureter sprang. It entered the bladder jointly with its homologue, but at that point it was dilated to such an extent that it encroached considerably on the lumen of the bladder. There was a left perinephric abscess.

Microscopically, the upper pole of the left kidney showed areas of dense sclerotic tissue within which are seen embryonal tubules surrounded by concentric rings of loose connective tissue. There is no inflammatory reaction in these areas. On the right the renal parenchyma showed no structural changes or inflammation (H & E, 60×). Other portions of the kidneys were not dysplastic.

179
HYDRONEPHROSIS. PARENCHYMAL ATROPHY

Male weighing 1,800 gm. Gestational age, 40 weeks. Admitted at 3 hours of life in respiratory distress. Chest x-rays were typical of pulmonary hyaline membrane disease. The infant died in respiratory arrest 6 hours after admission.

Histopathologic Examination. Gross examination revealed the presence of calyceal ectasia on the right. Large areas of parenchyma ap-

peared to have no structural detail. The left kidney was normal. Microscopically, it was apparent that a large portion of the right renal parenchyma was very atrophic, cortex as well as medulla. The cortex was reduced to a narrow rim in which isolated glomeruli persisted along with deeply basophilic tubules. Some papillae were totally sclerotic, lacking any tubular formations. Although some tubules showed an embryonal appearance, no other defects of differentiation were seen in the sections examined. Note the flattening of the papilla and loss of the calyceal contour. The pelvic epithelium is normal; there is no inflammatory infiltration (H & E, 60×).

Examination of the lung confirmed the diagnosis of atelectasis and pulmonary hyaline membranes.

180
SEGMENTAL ATROPHY

Female weighing 2,950 gm. Gestational age, 38 weeks. Clinical data are given with Figure 65.

Histopathologic Examination. The combined weight of the kidneys was 21 gm. Both showed areas of flattening on the surface.

Microscopic examination reveals two different types of renal cortex. On the left there is normal parenchyma penetrated by two medullary rays. On the right, with no intermediate transition, the cortical parenchyma shows obvious contraction, with sclerosis and atrophy of cortical elements, although some normal glomeruli persist. The corticomedullary junction is vague. The pelvis also shows marked sclerosis. There is no inflammatory infiltration (H & E, 60×).

None of the sections showed areas of dysplasia or cystic change. The histologic features that permit differentiation between segmental hypoplasia such as this and segmental dysplasia are the anomalous tissues, such as nests of cartilage or persistent elements that are inappropriate for the developmental age of the child. In segmental dysplasia an accessary ureter is often found in relation to the affected area.

Other findings: Anencephaly, agenesis of posterior lobe of the pituitary, bilateral adrenal hypoplasia, and necrotizing pneumonia (Fig. 65).

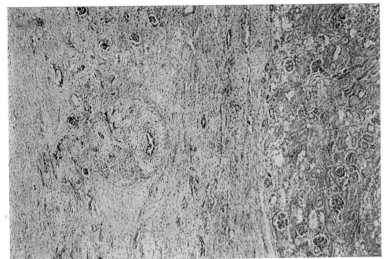

178

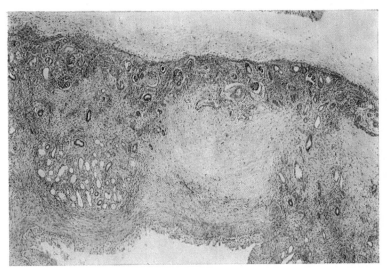

179

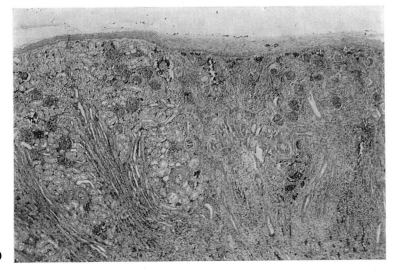

180

181
POLYCYSTIC KIDNEY. INFANTILE TYPE

Male weighing 3,000 gm. Unknown gestational age. Admitted 1 hour after delivery in moribund condition with gasping respirations, marked hypotonia, and extreme bradycardia. The facies was rather odd, and the ears were obviously low. The abdomen was very much distended; palpation revealed two large rounded masses, firm and movable, occupying each of the iliac fossae. Death occurred 40 minutes after admission.

Histopathologic Examination. The kidneys weighed 25 gm each. They occupied a considerable part of the abdominal cavity. The external appearance was reasonably normal save for the presence of minute cysts. On section, however, they showed a typically spongy appearance, the cavities being elongate.

Figure 181 shows transformation of the parenchyma into cystic cavities separated by loose connective tissue. In the most peripheral areas some glomeruli and tubules persist, the latter with immature characteristics. There was no inflammation or dysplasia (H & E, 60×).

Other findings: Bilateral pulmonary hypoplasia and cystic dysplasia of interlobular bile ducts. The pancreas was normal.

182
SUBCAPSULAR RENAL CYSTS

Male weighing 2,330 gm. Gestational age, 34 weeks. Admitted at 3 hours of life. In the next few hours a full-blown picture of intestinal obstruction developed and surgery was performed for the diagnosis of duodenal atresia. Three days later signs of respiratory insufficiency set in, accompanied by bouts of hypertonicity. Death occurred in respiratory arrest.

Histopathologic Examination. The kidneys weighed 28 and 12 gm respectively; the right showed multiple superficial cysts occupying about one third of the cortex. The left showed only an occasional cyst. There were no anomalies of the excretory pathways.

Microscopically, a cystic zone can be seen directly under the renal capsule. The cysts are small and are separated from one another by fibrous stroma. In the deeper portions of the cortex, scattered microcysts were visible (Masson, 60×). This type of lesion is frequently, though not exclusively, encountered in cases of obstruction of the lower excretory channels in the later stages of fetal development.

Other findings: Muscular defect in the anterior wall of the stomach, moderate aspiration of amniotic fluid, and extensive subarachnoid hemorrhage.

183
CACCHI-RICCI DISEASE. MEDULLARY CYSTIC KIDNEY

Female weighing 3,300 gm. Gestational age, 38 weeks. Admitted at 5 days of life because of a large umbilical hernia, cleft palate, and respiratory difficulty. On admission she exhibited hypotonia and hyporeflexia. Chest films indicated aspiration pneumonia. There was marked palpebral edema. Metabolic acidosis. Medium grade cardiomegaly. EEG tracing was abnormal, with irritative peaks in the right temporoparietal region. Cardiologic evaluation suggested hypoplasia of left chambers. The infant died 17 days after admission.

Histopathologic Examination. The kidneys were large, with a combined weight of 64 gm. On section, numerous cysts were apparent in the medullary zone. The corticomedullary junction was visible.

Figure 183 includes a portion of medulla showing cystic dilatation of distal and collecting tubules. The cysts are variable in size and some of them have irregular outlines. On the right there is a portion of cortex containing some normal glomeruli and an occasional dilated tubule (Masson, 60×).

Other findings: Polysegmented lungs with occasional hypoplastic lobules, foci of bronchopneumonia, preductal coarctation, hypoplasia of left heart chambers, and areas of dysplasia in the pancreas.

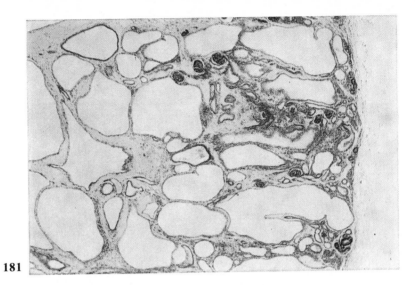

181

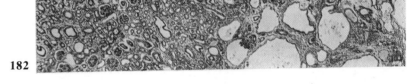

182

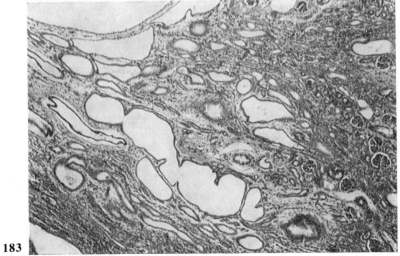

183

184
RENAL CYSTS IN CHROMOSOMAL ABNORMALITY

Male weighing 2,970 gm. Gestational age, 41 weeks. Admitted at 8 hours because of multiple congenital malformations. Examination suggested trisomy 13 with congenital cardiac anomaly; this was corroborated by karyotyping. Respiratory arrest occurred and the child was pronounced dead 48 hours after admission.

Histopathologic Examination. In our series of cases of trisomy 13 we have noticed the striking frequency of renal anomalies in the form of isolated glomerular and tubular microcysts unaccompanied by any important changes in renal architecture or any dysplastic lesions (Masson, 187.5×).

Other findings (aside from components of trisomy 13): Full-blown tetralogy of Fallot and extensive pulmonary atelectasis.

185
RENAL CYSTIC CLUSTERS

Male weighing 1,450 gm. Gestational age, 26 weeks. One of twins. Breech delivery followed by severe anoxia requiring intensive resuscitation. Admitted at 2 hours in a state that suggested imminent death. Cyanosis was deep, breathing was of gasping type, and chest films indicated pulmonary hyaline membrane disease. Death followed within an hour.

Histopathologic Examination. The kidneys were of average shape and weight for this age. Microscopically, in some areas of the cortex and especially in the subcapsular portions, there were clusters of cysts separated by fibrous tissue; some cysts contained remnants of glomeruli. The nephrogenic zone is visible in the left upper portion of the picture. There is also an occasional petechia in the deeper cortex (H & E, 60×).

Other findings: Alveolar pulmonary hemorrhages and early pulmonary hyaline membranes.

186
POLAR RENAL HYPOPLASIA

Female weighing 3,750 gm. Gestational age, 39 weeks. Apgar score 2 at birth. Admitted at 1 hour of life in grave general condition, with respiratory distress, pallor, hypotonia, and no response to stimuli. She died 30 minutes later despite aggressive resuscitation measures.

Histopathologic Examination. The kidneys weighed 30 gm together. Both showed obvious lobulation. In the lower pole of the left kidney the lobulations were small and very numerous.

Figure 186 shows a section of that zone. There is moderate atrophy of the parenchyma. Cystic cavities located both in the cortex and the medulla are quite conspicuous. In the subcapsular area, note the presence of a thick fibrous sheath around a tubule. There were no cartilaginous nests or embryonal tubules (Masson, 60×).

Other findings: Ruptured subcapsular hematoma of the liver with resulting hemoperitoneum, signs of anoxia, incompletely expanded lungs with areas of overaeration proximally.

187
MICROCYSTIC TUBULAR DYSPLASIA

Male weighing 3,600 gm, full term. At 20 days a picture resembling nephrotic syndrome developed. A renal biopsy was performed, and the specimen was submitted for study. No other data available.

Histopathologic Examination. The general architecture of the kidney is maintained, but the epithelium of the convoluted tubules is flattened and the lumina are dilated, forming small cysts of uniform size. The glomeruli show no significant changes. The interstitium and vessels are normal (H & E, 60×).

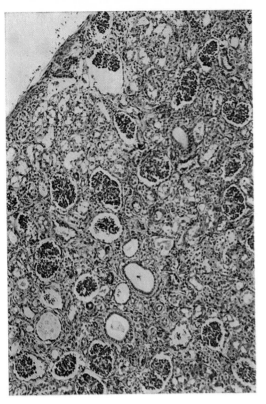

184

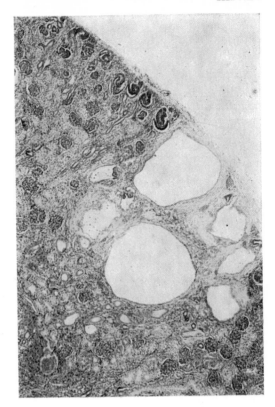

185

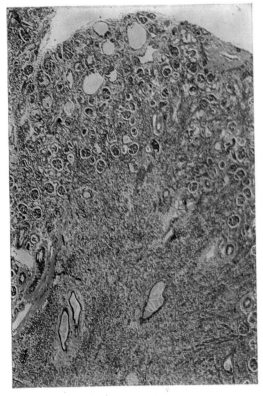

186

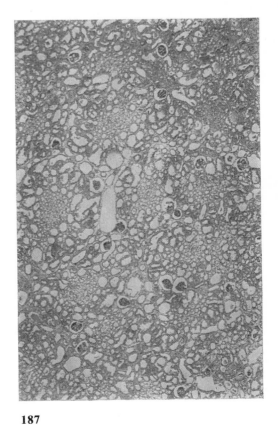

187

188/189/190/191
UNILATERAL RENAL NEPHROBLASTOMATOSIS IN A CASE OF TRIPLOIDY

Male weighing 2,430 gm. Gestational age, 40 weeks. Cesarean delivery. Giant placenta with mole-like changes. Admitted at 3 hours because of marked hypotonia, poor general condition, and severe bradycardia. Hydrocephalic appearance was striking, with a cranial perimeter of 38 cm. The root of the nose was depressed, the forehead was bulging, the interpupillary distance was increased, and there was microophthalmia with some exophthalmos. The ears were low. The following were also noted: lumbosacral myelomeningocele, bilateral undescended testes, underdeveloped penis, penoscrotal hypospadias, and bilateral clubfeet with partial syndactyly between the first and second toes. Radiographically, irregular ossification of the cranial vault was observed, and in both tarsal regions there were punctate images reminiscent of chondrodysplasia punctata. The child's general condition worsened rapidly, respirations became more and more labored, blood was expelled by mouth, and finally death occurred at 36 hours.

Cultures of blood, urine, and cerebrospinal fluid were all negative. Chromosome studies of peripheral blood demonstrated the presence of 69 chromosomes type 69 XXY. The parents' karyotypes were normal.

Histopathologic Examination. The weight of the kidneys was normal. The left showed a globular appearance of the upper pole. Microscopically, the right kidney was normal. In the left, the architecture was profoundly altered (Fig. 188, H & E, 60×). There are irregular collections of embryonal tubules set in densely cellular undifferentiated tissue, creating a pattern comparable to that of a Wilms' tumor (Fig. 189, H & E, 187.5×).

Figure 190 represents a sarcomatoid area (Masson, 375×).

Other areas of the renal cortex showed pericapsular glomerular fibrosis with partial hyalinization of the loop (Fig. 191, Masson, 375×). According to Nicholson, this type of tumor represents a deviation of renal development in which growth continues but differentiation is altered. This general disturbance of the metanephric blastema, with excessive proliferation, differs from other congenital disturbances such as renal cystic transformations in that the latter represent basically an arrest of proliferation.

It is obvious that among the "tumor" masses and even within them there are poorly organized and anomalous glomeruli and tubules. This indicates that differentiation of the blastemic areas is continuing. These poorly differentiated renal elements end up as regressive phenomena, with marked sclerosis of the glomeruli.

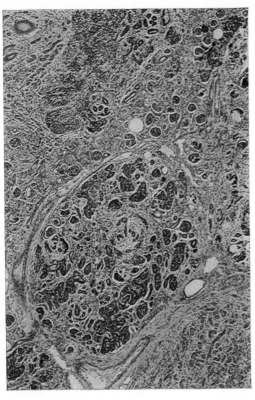

188

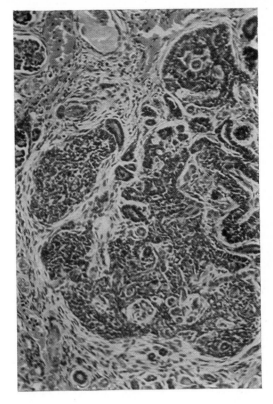

189

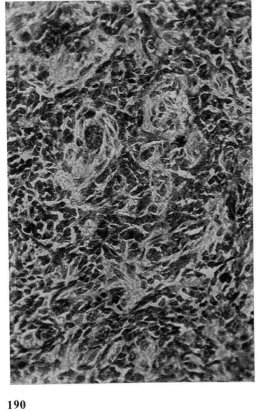

190

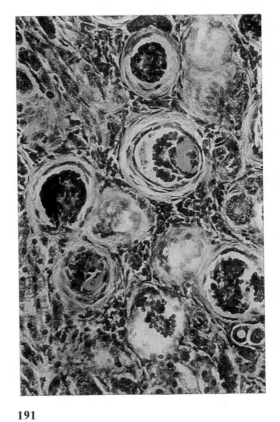

191

CORTICAL NECROSIS

Male weighing 4,500 gm. Admitted at 22 days of age because of sclerema in both lower extremities and abscesses at various locations.

For 5 days there had been fever, tachypnea, and diarrhea. On admission there was serious metabolic acidosis with pH of 6.86 and BE of −23 mEq/L. Blood culture was positive: 32 colonies of *Pyocyaneus* per milliliter of cultured blood. He died 3 days after admission.

Histopathologic Examination. Figure 192 shows extensive necrosis of the renal cortex, sparing only a thin subcapsular layer. The medulla and the juxtamedullary zone are preserved. In affected areas, the nuclei have disappeared, within both the tubules and the glomeruli, all of which are reduced to the status of eosinophilic "shadows." There is no inflammatory reaction. Small, intensely basophilic calcium deposits are also in evidence (H & E, 60×).

Other findings: Bronchopneumonia, septic foci in various organs, and fatty degeneration of the liver.

RENAL TUBULAR NECROSIS

Male weighing 4,400 gm. Gestational age, 40 weeks. Apgar score 2 at birth, requiring energetic resuscitation. Admitted at 1 hour of life in poor condition, with respiratory difficulties, pallor, and hepatosplenomegaly. Studies showed Rh isommunization, with a positive direct Coombs reaction. After treatment of the existing acidosis, an exchange transfusion was carried out. Death occurred 18 hours after admission.

Histopathologic Examination. The proximal convoluted tubules show signs of acute necrosis characterized by lysis of the nuclear chromatin and cytoplasmic acidophilia. Note the normal appearance of the glomeruli and the tubuli recti (H & E, 187.5×).

Other findings: Considerable extramedullary hematopoiesis in liver and spleen, abundant subarachnoid hemorrhage, and petechiae in thymus and myocardium.

HEMORRHAGIC INFARCTION OF KIDNEY

Male weighing 3,760 gm. Gestational age, 40 weeks. Admitted at 16 hours of age in poor general condition, with marked pallor, hypotonia, weak cry, signs of collapse, and systolic murmur. Four centimeter hepatomegaly. Microhematocrit, 18 per cent. Severe metabolic acidosis. The acidosis was corrected, and a transfusion was given. Radiographic studies and paracentesis established a diagnosis of hemoperitoneum, possibly the result of rupture of the liver. This was confirmed at surgery. More details are given in comments on Figure 246.

Histopathologic Examination. Necrosis of renal parenchyma is associated with hemorrhagic infiltration of the interstitium. Glomerular capillaries are engorged. The glomerulus seen at the upper left in Figure 194 shows early signs of necrosis manifested by pyknosis of the nuclei (H & E, 375×).

For other findings see Figure 246.

BRAIN TISSUE EMBOLISM IN THE KIDNEY

Male weighing 1,000 gm. Gestational age, 28 weeks. Apgar score 5 at birth. This case was described with Figure 104 in connection with brain tissue embolism in a pulmonary vessel.

Histopathologic Examination. Figure 195 shows an arcuate artery that is distended with brain tissue; the latter contains small vessels (H & E, 375×). Similar emboli were seen in pulmonary vessels (Fig. 104).

Other findings: Subdural hemorrhage, focal subarachnoid hemorrhages, and general visceral immaturity.

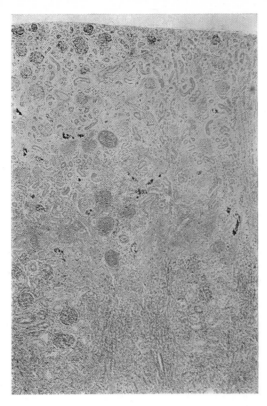

192

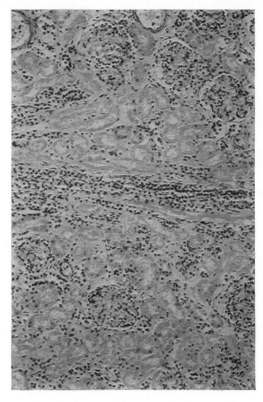

193

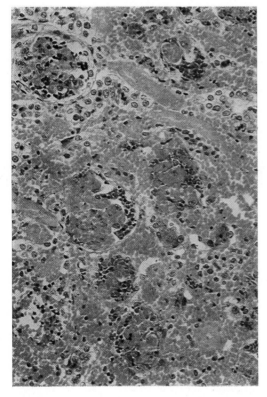

194

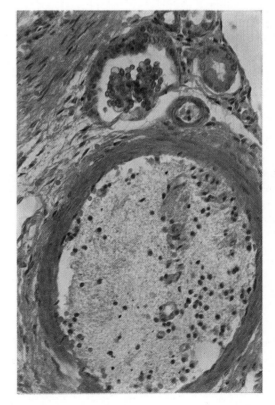

195

196
RENAL LISTERIOMA

Male weighing 1,200 gm. Gestational age, 30 weeks. Data are given with Figure 64.

Histopathologic Examination. At the center of Figure 196 a nodular inflammatory lesion can be seen, consisting mainly of mononuclear cells. There is no necrosis. The borders between the lesion and the adjacent parenchyma are sharp. (Masson, 187.5×).

With appropriate staining methods it was possible to demonstrate clusters of gram-positive organisms that were argyrophilic by the Levaditi technique.

Similar granulomas were observed in the lung (Fig. 64), liver, and spleen.

197
CYTOMEGALIC INCLUSION NEPHRITIS

Male weighing 2,700 gm. Unknown gestational age. Apgar score 3 at birth, requiring strenuous resuscitation. Admitted 1 hour later in poor general condition with mild cyanosis, moderate respiratory difficulty, two fingerbreadth hepatomegaly, tachycardia, and striking green discoloration of the umbilical cord. Chest x-ray showed reduced lung fields, diaphragm at the level of the fifth interspace. pH 6.9, pCO_2 78 mm Hg, BE −20 mEq/L. Ten per cent dextrose and 1 M bicarbonate were started intravenously. Subsequently the respiratory signs were intensified, and mixed metabolic and respiratory acidosis continued. Death occurred 24 hours after admission. There was no purpura.

Histopathologic Examination. Figure 197 shows a renal tubule. Some of its cells show a nuclear basophilic inclusion surrounded by a clear halo; the nuclear chromatin is displaced peripherally (H & E, 375×).

Around that tubule there is marked inflammatory infiltration consisting mostly of round mononuclear cells. Other tubules contained inclusions without inflammatory reaction.

Other findings: Cells with cytomegalic inclusions in the lung without inflammatory reaction, left pulmonary hypoplasia, and focal subarachnoid hemorrhage.

198
ACUTE PYELONEPHRITIS

Male weighing 3,100 gm. Unknown gestational age. Admitted at 13 days of life. Same case as Figure 77.

Histopathologic Examination. There were no gross malformations of the urinary tract. The kidneys showed many abscesses. Figure 198 shows a small abscess with surrounding histiocytic reaction. The collecting tubules are dilated; the epithelium is flattened and partly desquamated, and the lumen contains many granulocytes. The stroma is loose and also infiltrated by polymorphonuclear leukocytes (H & E, 187.5×).

Both lungs showed interstitial pneumonitis (Fig. 77).

199
GLOMERULAR THROMBOCAPILLARITIS IN ENDOTOXIC SHOCK

Male weighing 3,400 gm. Unknown gestational age. Admitted at 16 days of life. For 6 days there had been discharge from the left ear and he had refused to nurse. Three days before admission jaundice appeared; the right ear began to drain, and left facial paralysis became manifest.

In addition, examination disclosed hepatomegaly and metabolic acidosis. Studies showed: 22,400 wbc/ml, SGOT 680 u/L, SGPT 290 u/L, bilirubin 6.2 mg/100 ml, albuminuria. Cultures of gastric contents and ear discharge positive for *E. coli;* blood culture negative.

Urine culture produced 250,000 colonies of *E. coli* per milliliter of urine. In the next 3 days the general septic picture became worse, and the child died in circulatory collapse.

Histopathologic Examination. In the glomerulus shown in Figure 199 there are intensely acidophilic hyaline thrombi. The endothelial cells are swollen. The lining cells of the neighboring renal tubules show cloudy swelling (H & E, 600×).

Autopsy demonstrated the presence of generalized sepsis manifested by multiple necrotizing granulomas, especially in the liver and myocardium.

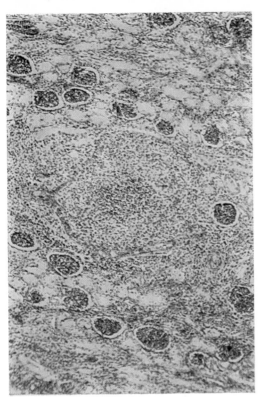

196

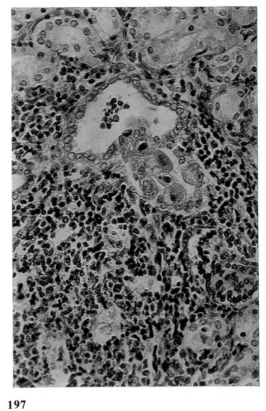

197

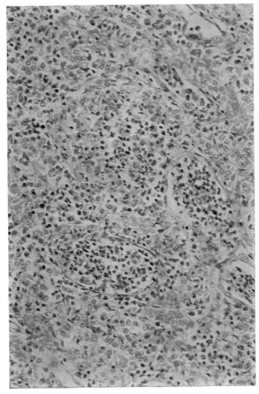

198

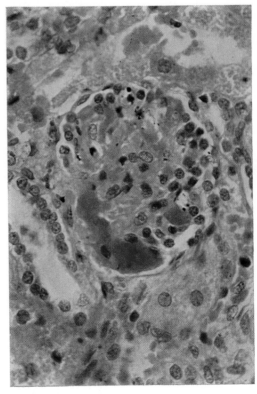

199

200
THROMBOSIS OF ARCUATE VEIN

Female weighing 3,420 gm. Gestational age, 38 weeks. Jaundice due to anti-A incompatibility had responded well to exchange transfusion. At 15 days of life, diarrhea and respiratory difficulty developed, necessitating admission. There were poor general condition, intercostal retraction, tachypnea, hypertonic type of dehydration. pH 7.06, pCO_2 31 mm Hg, BE -22 mEq/L, microhematocrit 43 per cent, Hb. 17 gm/100 ml. In spite of treatment, the infant died 28 hours after admission.

Histopathologic Examination. Grossly, the kidneys appeared congested, with hemorrhagic areas. Both renal veins were patent. Microscopically, many vessels at the corticomedullary junction showed occlusion caused by fibrinoleukocytic thrombi such as the one shown in Figure 200. The surrounding renal parenchyma is markedly congested (H & E, 60×).

Other findings: Large bilateral foci of bronchopneumonia and bilateral adrenal hemorrhagic foci.

201
RENAL PAPILLITIS

Male weighing 3,000 gm. Gestational age, 38 weeks. Admitted at 6 days of life with a 2 day history of jaundice and a convulsion the day before. There was poor general condition with marked hypotonia, deep jaundice, and persistent caput (cephalhematoma). Isoimmunization was ruled out by pertinent studies. Glucose 6-phosphate-dehydrogenase was within normal limits. Total bilirubin, 23.4 mg/100 ml. Leukocytosis 18,400 wbc/ml. Negative blood culture. Exchange transfusion was carried out. Spinal tap yielded clear fluid under increased pressure, with no abnormal elements. Death occurred 20 hours after admission.

Histopathologic Examination. Microscopically, there was marked engorgement of small vessels in the renal papilla. At the center of Figure 201 there is a large nongranulomatous focus of granulocytic infiltration (Masson, 187.5×).

The autopsy revealed scattered microabscesses in the liver, edema of the brain, and no bile-staining of the basal ganglia. There was vacuolar degeneration of the renal tubular cells.

202
RENAL EXTRAMEDULLARY HEMATOPOIESIS

Male weighing 2,030 gm. Gestational age, 34 weeks. Admitted 1 hour after delivery and remained for 2 weeks with an uneventful course. He was discharged weighing 2,650 gm and in good health.

Readmitted 10 days later with diarrhea and severe dehydration. The appearance was that of general sepsis, with depressed sensorium, pallor, serious metabolic acidosis, abdominal distention, and gasping respirations. Blood culture was positive for *Pseudomonas*. He died 24 hours after admission.

Histopathologic Examination. At the corticomedullary junction there are poorly defined foci of hematopoietic tissue (H & E, 375×). There were neither polymorphonuclear infiltrates nor granulomas. This type of lesion is frequently found in premature infants who later become septic. We have observed similar foci in myeloproliferative syndromes.

Other autopsy findings included the presence of a small number of microabscesses in the liver together with intracellular cholestasis and occasional bile thrombi. Capillaries of the alveolar septa in the lung contained many polymorphonuclear leukocytes.

203
IDIOPATHIC CONGENITAL NEPHROTIC SYNDROME

Female weighing 3,050 gm. Unknown gestational age. Admitted 23 days after birth because of generalized edema and pallor. On admission her general condition was fair; pallor and generalized edema were pronounced in the face. In the preceding 24 hours she had gained 250 gm in weight. There was albuminuria to the extent of 4 gm/L. There were no abnormal elements in the urine. Total protein was 54 gm/L (5.4 gm/100 ml). Albumin 7.62 gm/100 ml; alpha 1 globulin 1.99, alpha 2 globulin 32.43, beta globulin 6.91, and gamma globulin 5.73 mg/100 ml; and blood urea, 32 mg/100 ml. Total lipids 1,010 mg/100 ml. Cholesterol 458 mg/100 ml. The diagnosis of idiopathic congenital nephrotic syndrome was made. Renal biopsy was performed.

Histopathologic Examination. The renal architecture is normal. The renal tubules show no anomalies. The glomerulus illustrated in Figure 203 is moderately cellular especially as regards the mesangium. There is an obvious tendency to glomerular lobulation (Masson, 600×).

Reticulum and PAS stains did not reveal any changes in the basement membranes.

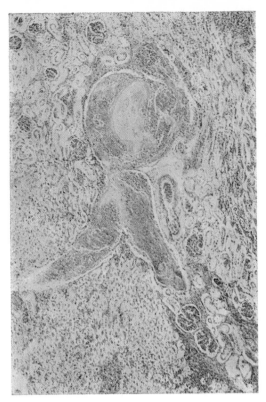

200

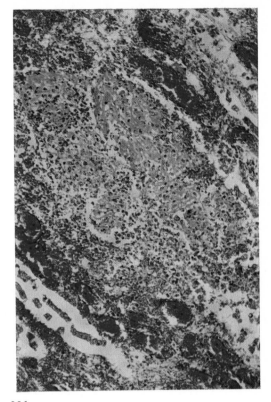

201

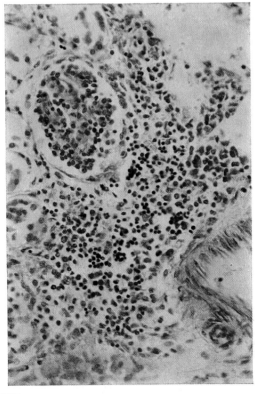

202

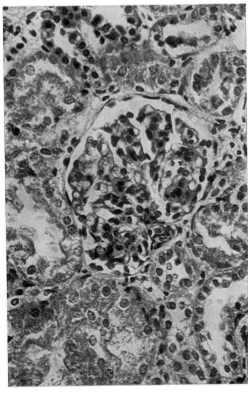

203

Digestive Tract

204
CONGENITAL EPULIS (GRANULAR CELL TUMOR)

Male weighing 3,500 gm. Gestational age, 44 weeks. Normal delivery.

Admitted 2 days after birth because of a pedunculated nodule the size of a cherry, attached to the right lower gum. It was excised.

Histopathologic Examination. The gingival tumor is made up of large round or polygonal cells with small central nuclei and granular eosinophilic cytoplasm (H & E, 375×).

The epithelial surface of the mucosa has a straight lower border without any ridges. In some areas there are cords of epithelial odontogenic cells. The relationship between congenital epulis and the granular cell myoblastoma that appears in later life is debatable. In the latter there is usually pseudoepitheliomatous hyperplasia of the surface epithelium, especially in tumors located in the tongue, and there are no related odontogenic remnants.

205
MUCUS-SECRETING CYST OF THE TONGUE

Female weighing 4,400 gm. Born at 40 weeks of gestation. Normal delivery. Apgar score 10. Physical examination on admission was normal except for the presence of a nodule the size of a walnut on the ventral aspect of the tongue in the midline.

Forty-eight hours after admission the cystic mass was excised by way of a ventral approach. The postoperative course was completely satisfactory, and she was released 10 days later.

Histopathologic Examination. The cystic structure shows an epithelial lining made up of goblet cells. Peripheral to that there is a band of fibrous connective tissue that outlines the cyst and separates it from the muscular tissue of the tongue. In contrast to the duplication cyst shown in Figure 206, there is no smooth muscle in the wall (H & E, 187.5×).

Unlike retention cysts such as this, mucoceles represent pseudocystic accumulations of mucinous material without any epithelial lining.

206
HETEROTOPIC LINGUAL CYSTS

Female weighing 4,400 gm. Gestational age, 42 weeks. No significant data regarding the immediate neonatal period.

The infant came to the hospital at 15 days of age because of the presence, since birth, of a lump in the base of the tongue the size of a hazel nut. Two days after admission this soft tumor was excised from within the deep tissues of the tongue.

Histopathologic Examination. The cyst is lined by pseudostratified ciliated columnar epithelium that includes a few goblet cells. In some areas it is replaced by stratified squamous epithelium. The lesion is interpreted as a type of duplication (esophageal?) because of the presence in its wall of a double layer of smooth muscle, one stratum longitudinal and the other circular, the inner one being conspicuously thick. In the lower part of the photograph there is a layer of striated muscle corresponding to the musculature of the tongue (Masson 60×).

207
PAROTID CYTOMEGALIC INCLUSION DISEASE

Female weighing 3,140 gm. Gestational age, 38 weeks. Admitted 12 hours after birth for serious respiratory insufficiency. Among the important data there was the history of serious neonatal asphyxia that had required resuscitation. The amniotic fluid had been stained with meconium.

On admission the infant had rapid respirations, cyanosis, intercostal retraction, a weak cry, and hypotonia. Aspiration of gastric contents yielded 50 ml of a greenish yellow fluid. Chest x-ray showed changes very suggestive of aspiration, predominantly in the right lung field. There was mixed acidosis: pH 7.19, pCO_2 60.5 mm Hg, BE −9.5 mEq/L. Crises of apnea continued in spite of intensive treatment. The infant died 18 hours after admission.

Histopathologic Examination. The epithelial lining of the glandular structure in the center of Figure 207 contains six large cells with huge nuclei, each surrounded by a clear halo and with granular cytoplasm (Masson, 600×).

There was no inflammatory reaction, and there were no cytomegalic inclusions in other organs.

Autopsy revealed necrotizing granulocytic pneumonia with massive aspiration of amniotic debris.

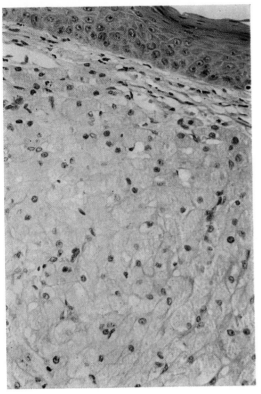

204

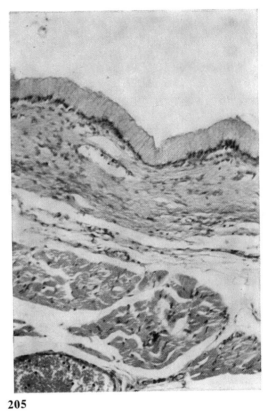

205

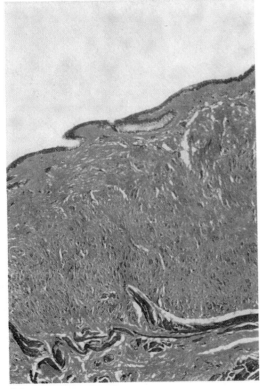

206

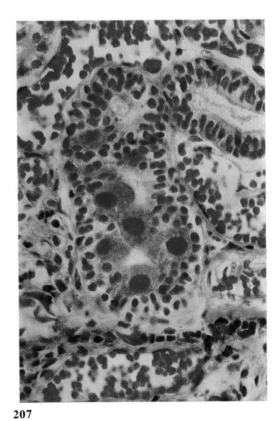

207

208
SUPPURATIVE PAROTITIS

Male weighing 2,000 gm. Gestational age, 32 weeks. Born by breech delivery. Apgar score 2 at birth, requiring intensive resuscitation. Large hematomas in the buttocks and over the left hip. Admitted at 3 hours of life in very poor general condition with loss of tone, intercostal retraction, weak cry, tachypnea, and striking pallor. There was marked cyanosis in both lower extremities. Microhematocrit 19 per cent, hemoglobin 8.05 gm/100 ml. There were periods of hypertonicity alternating with the prevailing loss of tone. Spinal tap yielded hemorrhagic fluid. Blood transfusion was carried out. EEG showed poorly integrated bioelectric cerebral activity with flattened waves. Echoencephalogram was normal. There was no shift of the midline. Three days after admission sclerema of the lower jaw and anterior aspect of the neck appeared, together with firm induration and bluish discoloration of the left parotid region. The infant's general condition worsened progressively, with respiratory failure and episodes of generalized hypertonicity.

Histopathologic Examination. The parotid tissue is extensively necrotic. The area shown in Figure 208 shows no well-preserved acini but rather severe polymorphonuclear leukocytic inflammatory infiltration. The more basophilic irregular areas represent accumulations of bacteria (H & E, 375×).

At autopsy there was also a supratentorial cerebral hemorrhage, fibrinoleukocytic bronchopneumonia, lymphoid depletion of the thymus, and a hemorrhagic renal infarct.

209
HEMANGIOMA OF THE PAROTID

Twenty-eight day old male weighing 8,000 gm. Delivery normal. No significant history. Normal nutrition. Brought to the dispensary because a right parotid mass had been present for 5 days.

The mass occupied the region of the ascending ramus of the mandible; it was soft and poorly outlined. It disappeared almost completely under direct pressure. The skin over it was light blue. Sialography and arteriography led to the preoperative diagnosis of hemangioma of the parotid, confirmed at surgery.

The external carotid and jugular vessels had to be ligated because they were directly involved in the mass and lay beneath it. The tumor and associated parotid lobules were excised successfully and without further event.

Histopathologic Examination. Figure 209 shows disruption of parotid gland architecture by neoplastic tissue composed of angioblastic cells without lumina and delicate capillary clefts lined by uniform endothelium. In the midst of this tissue are a number of excretory ducts and a group of acinar cells (H & E, 375×).

210
IMMATURE ESOPHAGUS

Male weighing 3,800 gm. Gestational age, 40 weeks. Delivery involved fetal anoxia. Apgar score 1 at birth, requiring intensive resuscitation. At 1 hour of age the infant was admitted in very poor condition with generalized hypotonia with areflexia, absence of spontaneous movement, generalized cyanosis, shallow breathing, and livid spots on the chest. Intensive treatment failed, and the infant died in 4 hours.

Histopathologic Examination. In some sections of the esophagus the normal stratified epithelium is covered by a single layer of ciliated columnar cells with abundant eosinophilic cytoplasm. There is also marked congestion of vessels in the corium (H & E, 600 ×).

Another finding at autopsy was the presence of numerous foci of hematopoiesis in the liver. This is unusual in an infant born at term and of adequate body weight.

At autopsy there was complete pulmonary anectasia and an incidental small neuroblastoma in one adrenal.

211
HEMORRHAGE IN THE ESOPHAGUS

Female weighing 1,060 gm. Gestational age, 25 weeks. Apgar score 4 at birth. Admitted at 1 hour of life in poor general condition with cyanosis, hypotonia, and generalized edema. Microhematocrit 67 per cent, pH 7.08, pCO_2 65 mm Hg, BE, −11.5 mEq/L. In spite of treatment with correction of acidosis, episodes of apnea recurred repeatedly, and she died 6 hours later.

Histopathologic Examination. The epithelium of the esphagus is well preserved, while in the submucosa there is extensive hemorrhagic infiltration. The smooth muscle bundles are separated by edema with the admixture of some erythrocytes (H & E, 187.5×).

Autopsy further disclosed the presence of hemoperitoneum (due to the rupture of a subcapsular hematoma of the liver); petechiae in the lung, thymus, and liver; pulmonary atelectasis with focal bronchopneumonia; and generalized evidences of immaturity.

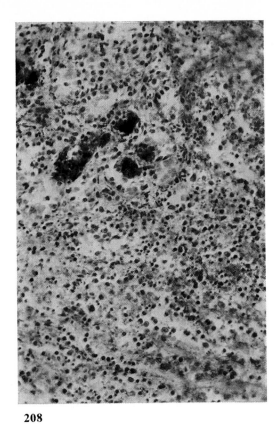

208

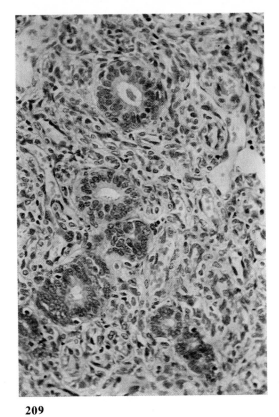

209

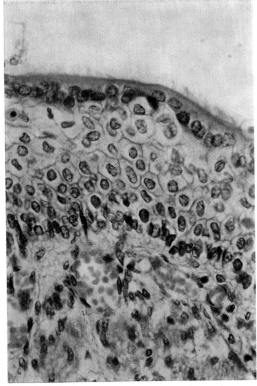

210

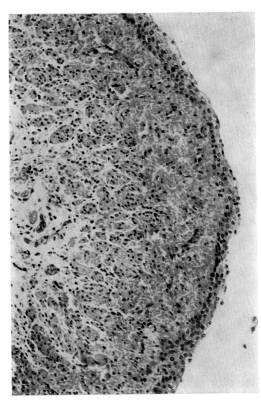

211

212
EROSIVE EOSPHAGITIS

Male weighing 2,800 gm, born at term. This is the same case as is illustrated in Figures 128, 129, and 217.

Histopathologic Examination. Figure 212 shows a section of the distal esophagus. The surface epithelium has disappeared; small remnants remain visible only in the upper right corner of the illustration. The superficial lamina propria is infiltrated by inflammatory cells and erythrocytes. There are some seromucinous glands in the submucosa (H & E, 60×).

A polyethylene gastric tube had been in place and had been changed every 48 hours. Furthermore, gastric aspiration had been carried out as part of resuscitation at birth.

At autopsy there was suppurative bronchopneumonia with a substantial hemorrhagic component; multiple foci of necrosis of the myocardium (Figs. 128 and 129), large areas of hemorrhagic necrosis of the intestinal mucosa (Fig. 217), and foci of encephalomalacia were also seen.

213
CYTOMEGALIC INCLUSION DISEASE OF THE ESOPHAGUS

Female weighing 11,050 gm. Gestational age, 29 weeks. This same case is illustrated in Figure 229, cytomegalic inclusion disease involving the pancreatic islets.

Histopathologic Examination. In the superficial portion of the corium of the esophagus two cells can be seen containing small basophilic intranuclear inclusions, accompanied by a scanty inflammatory round cell infiltrate. The vessels are engorged (H & E, 375×).

There were typical cytomegalic cells in other organs, particularly the liver.

214
CANDIDA ESOPHAGITIS

Female weighing 1,040 gm. Gestational age, 27 weeks. Vertex presentation. Crisis of anoxia at birth.

Admitted 6 hours after birth as an immature infant in poor general condition with cyanosis, edema of the lower extremities, and hypotonia. The impression was one of generalized sepsis.

Appropriate therapeutic measures were undertaken, but the infant's general condition worsened. Blood culture was negative. On the third day of life, vomiting of bile-stained fluid occurred together with episodes of apnea and cyanosis. X-rays of the chest showed confluent nodular pulmonary infiltrates in both lung fields. In the last 2 days of life, diarrhea developed. Death occurred on the fifth day of life during an apneic episode.

Histopathologic Examination. The esophagus shows areas of epithelial erosion and accumulation of inflammatory elements and spores and hyphae of *Candida albicans* stained black by Gomori's methenamine silver method (375 ×).

At autopsy, necrotizing bronchopneumonia and *Candida* enteritis were also found.

215
HERPES ESOPHAGITIS

Male weighing 2,850 gm. Gestational age unknown. Admitted at 7 days of age for rejection of feedings of 2 days' duration and generally depressed condition with weak cry. On admission, he was mildly cyanotic. Rough systolic murmur at the apex. X-ray of the chest showed a heart of normal size. Electrocardiogram revealed no significant change save for a right-sided predominance, which is normal at this age. There was no significant hepatosplenomegaly, and the blood count, urinalysis, acid-base balance, and electrolytes were all within normal limits. Thirty-six hours after admission, the patient's condition deteriorated suddenly, with tachypnea and marked intercostal retraction. The infant died in respiratory arrest.

Histopathologic Examination. In the esophagus there are areas like that shown in Figure 215, with desquamation of epithelium and extensive ares of necrosis involving a considerable part of the lamina propria with cells containing eosinophilic inclusion bodies. The absence of any inflammatory infiltrate is noteworthy (H & E, 187.5×).

At autopsy the liver showed multiple punctate yellow lesions of pinhead size, uniformly scattered throughout the parenchyma. Microscopic examination showed these to be miliary foci of necrosis (Figs. 278 and 279); similar lesions were also found in the adrenals (Figs. 312 and 313), and there was interstitial pneumonia with hemorrhagic foci.

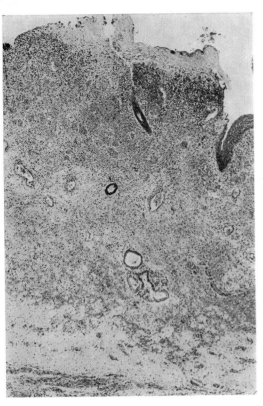

212

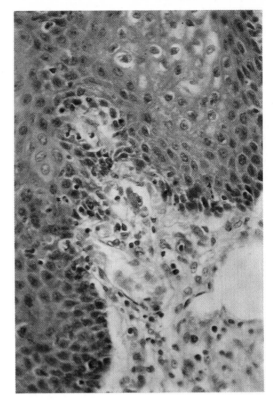

213

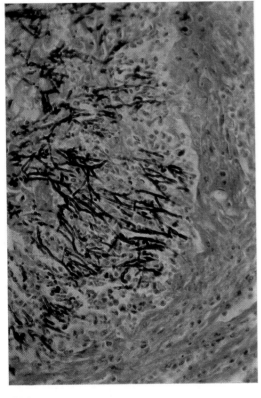

214

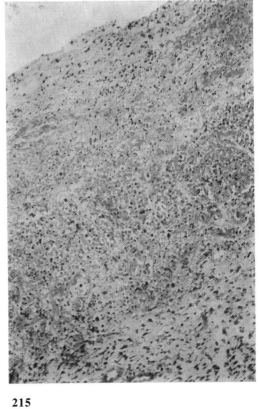

215

216
ACUTE GASTRIC ULCER

Female weighing 2,700 gm. Gestational age unknown.

Admitted 2 hours after birth in poor condition with generalized cyanosis, expiratory wheezing, microophthalmia, low placement of ears, tachycardia, enlargement of the liver, hypotonia, diminished reflexes, edema of extremities, and severe metabolic acidosis. Bicarbonate and 10 per cent dextrose solution were administered intravenously. In an x-ray of the chest, symmetrical enlargement of the heart was observed as well as extensive areas of diminished aeration in both lungs. At 3 days of age the infant experienced massive pulmonary hemorrhage with expulsion of abundant hemorrhagic and mucoid secretions from the upper airway. Respiratory arrest responded to resuscitation and assisted respiration. Twenty-four hours later, however, the child died.

Histopathologic Examination. Figure 216 shows an area of desquamation of the gastric mucosa with a shallow ulcer niche with a fibrinous and leukocytic covering lying on the base. Granulation tissue such as is seen in chronic peptic ulcers is not observed (Masson, 15 ×).

At autopsy there were also focal cerebral hemorrhages and massive bilateral pulmonary hemorrhage.

217
NECROTIZING ENTEROCOLITIS, EARLY STAGE

Male weighing 2,800 gm. Gestational age, 40 weeks. Same case as is illustrated in Figure 212, erosive esophagitis.

Histopathologic Examination. Figure 217 shows a segment of small bowel with necrosis and hemorrhage involving the superficial portion of the mucosa. The deeper portions are not affected, and similarly the muscularis mucosae and the submucosa are uninvolved (H & E, 187.5×).

Autopsy also showed suppurative bronchopneumonia with a conspicuous hemorrhagic component, multiple areas of myocardial necrosis (Figs. 128 and 129), encephalomalacia, and erosive esophagitis (Fig. 212).

218
NECROTIZING ENTEROCOLITIS, ADVANCED STAGE

Female weighing 840 gm. Gestational age unknown. This case was illustrated in Figure 234, focal pancreatic microdysplasia.

Histopathologic Examination. The intestinal mucosa shows extensive necrobiosis with superficial hemorrhagic foci. There is acute inflammatory infiltration especially in the submucosa. Some of the vessels contain hyaline thrombi (H & E, 187.5 ×).

Autopsy also demonstrated focal pulmonary hemorrhages and peritonitis, the result of intestinal perforation, in addition to focal pancreatic microdysplasia (Fig. 234).

219
PNEUMATOSIS CYSTOIDES INTESTINALIS

Sixteen hundred and thirty gram male born of a twin delivery. Gestational age, 32 weeks. Apgar score 4 at birth, requiring resuscitation. Admitted 24 hours later with decreased tone and jaundice. The following day a bout of gastrointestinal upset was accompanied by severe metabolic acidosis, distention of the abdomen, and bile-stained vomiting. There was deep jaundice with a total bilirubin of 18.4 mg/100 ml. No evidence of isoimmunization. Plain films of the abdomen showed dilated loops of small bowel without air-filled levels. The gastrointestinal picture worsened, and serious dehydration developed. Death occurred 24 hours later in cardiocirculatory failure.

Histopathologic Examination. Figure 219 shows marked cystic dilatation of the lymphatics of the intestinal wall, particularly in the submucosa. The giant cell reaction seen in pneumatosis cystoides intestinalis of the adult is not present (H & E, 15×).

The mesenteric lymph nodes also showed the picture of cystoid adenitis (cf. Fig. 348).

Autopsy revealed no significant pulmonary or cerebral lesions. There was fibrinous peritonitis. Extensive zones of hemorrhagic infiltration were found in the small bowel, and in some of them there was obvious necrotizing enteritis.

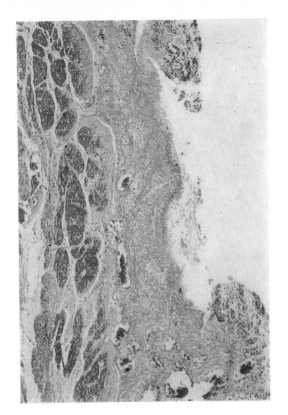

216

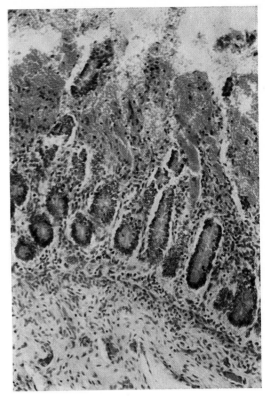

217

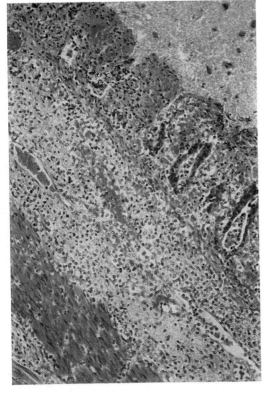

218

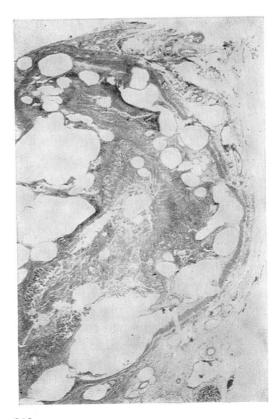

219

220
VOLVULUS WITH HEMORRHAGIC INFARCTION OF THE SMALL BOWEL

Female weighing 2,250 gm. Gestational age, 39 weeks. Normal delivery. Apgar score 10 at birth. Admitted 1 hour after birth. Physical examination on admission: essentially normal. Twenty-four hours later vomiting of bile-stained material. Two hours after that, bleeding by rectum occurred with marked abdominal distention, repeated vomiting of bile-stained material, and generally poor condition. Plain films of the abdomen showed an extensive area of the right hemiabdomen that appeared to contain no air. On the left side the intestinal loops were dilated without air-fluid levels.

Surgery was performed and volvulus was encountered. The terminal portion of the ileum had twisted twice on its axis; gangrene involved 15 cm of ileum. There was adhesive peritonitis. The gangrenous segment was resected, and an end-to-end anastomosis created. Two weeks later the child was discharged in satisfactory condition.

Histopathologic Examination. The wall of the resected intestine is frankly necrotic and shows diffuse hemorrhagic infiltration. The glandular pattern of the mucosa has disappeared completely, and the serosa is thickened by acute inflammatory infiltration (H & E, 60 ×).

221
INTRAUTERINE MECONIUM PERITONITIS

Female weighing 1,700 gm. Gestational age, 32 weeks. Breech delivery. Apgar score 2 at birth, requiring energetic resuscitation. Admitted at 2 hours of life in very poor general condition with generalized cyanosis, edema of the buttocks and lower extremities, hypotonia, moderate respiratory distress, and mixed acidosis. Subsequently, bouts of apnea required further resuscitatory maneuvers, and assisted respiration was instituted. The abdomen remained soft and pliable and the infant passed meconium twice. She died at 26 hours of age.

Histopathologic Examination. Figure 221 shows a section of thickened peritoneum in which are embedded basophilic amniotic squames as well as some calcific granules. There is no inflammatory infiltration (H & E, 600 ×).

Other findings: Disseminated petechiae, especially in the thymus and the myocardium, pulmonary anectasia, general immaturity, and mild dilatation of isolated pancreatic acini.

222
NEONATAL PERITONITIS

Female weighing 1,370 gm. Gestational age, 35 weeks. Admitted at 1 hour of life with some respiratory distress and generalized cyanosis. The radiographic findings were suspicious of aspiration of amniotic fluid, especially in the lower right lung field. The sensorium was depressed, but the abdomen seemed normal. Under standard measures of care the infant improved. At 48 hours, however, respiratory arrests necessitated repeated efforts at resuscitation. One of these bouts on the third hospital day was irreversible.

Histopathologic Examination. Autopsy disclosed gangrene of the bowel with perforation. Figure 222 shows a section of bowel. The serosa is markedly thickened and infiltrated by leukocytes mingled with cellular debris. Over the peritoneal surface there is a layer of fibrin (H & E, 375 ×).

Other findings: General immaturity, anoxic lesions, extensive pulmonary atelectasis, and signs of aspiration of meconium.

223
AGANGLIONIC MEGACOLON

Male weighing 4,500 gm. Normal delivery. Admitted at 28 days suffering from constipation from birth, with repeated bouts of near-obstruction. The abdomen was markedly distended and showed supplementary venous circulation. No masses were palpable. Rectal examination revealed an empty ampulla. X-rays demonstrated megacolon and megabladder. A Rehbein surgical procedure was carried out. The postoperative course was uneventful.

Histopathologic Examination. Sections of the resected stenotic portion of colon showed absence of ganglion cells. Figure 223 represents the junction of the two main muscular layers (longitudinal and circular). There is moderate hypertrophy of the myenteric plexus and absence of ganglion cells (H & E, 187.5 ×).

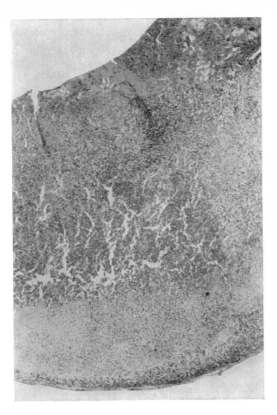

220

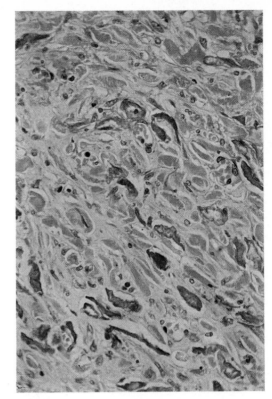

221

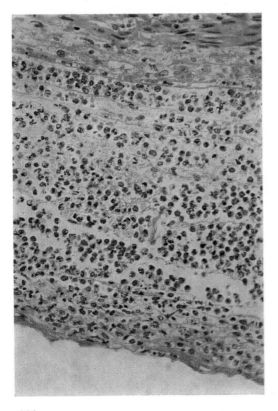

222

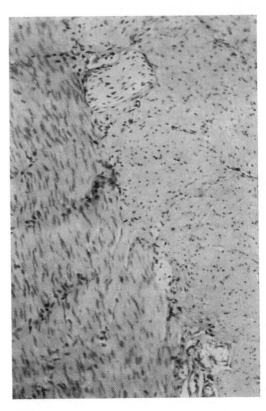

223

Pancreas

224

HEMATOPOIETIC ACTIVITY IN THE PANCREAS

Female weighing 2,000 gm. Gestational age, 35 weeks. Delivered in cephalic presentation 20 days after rupture of the membranes. Admitted 7 hours later with respiratory difficulty. On examination: Mongoloid features, hypotonia, some respiratory distress. X-rays of the chest suggested pulmonary hyaline membrane disease. Abdominal films showed a distribution of air shadows compatible with duodenal atresia. The respiratory picture worsened. Mixed acidosis was severe. She died at 30 hours following multiple bouts of apnea. Karyotyping showed trisomy 21.

Histopathologic Examination. The pancreatic stroma is densely infiltrated by hematopoietic elements. This form of extramedullary hematopoiesis is commonly seen in erythroblastosis, but may be observed in other processes (H & E, 375×).

Other findings: Duodenal atresia, pulmonary atelectasis, and pulmonary hyaline membranes.

225

METASTATIC NEUROBLASTOMA IN PANCREAS

Male weighing 3,250 gm. Gestational age, 39 weeks. Cesarean delivery. Admitted at 2 hours of life in serious condition, with marked pallor, absence of spontaneous movements, grunting, respiratory distress, bulging abdomen, and a gigantic palpable abdominal mass. More clinical details accompanying Figures 296 and 297.

Histopathologic Examination. The pancreatic interstitial stroma is infiltrated by cords of cells with dark-staining nuclei and very scanty cytoplasm. No changes can be seen in the acini (H & E, 375 ×).

Other findings: Bilateral adrenal neuroblastoma with involvement of the liver and pancreatic metastases, subtentorial hemorrhage.

226

LEUKEMIC INFILTRATION OF THE PANCREAS

Female weighing 3,200 gm. Gestational age, 38 weeks. One previous sibling had Down's syndrome and congenital heart disease.

This infant was admitted at 3 hours of life with generalized pallor, scattered hematomas and petechiae, nosebleed, respiratory distress, blowing apical systolic murmur, and hepatosplenomegaly.

Microhematocrit 19 per cent, Hb 7 gm/100 ml, platelets 30,000/cu mm, leukocytes 118,000/cu mm, 68 per cent of which were immature cells resembling lymphocytes while the other 32 per cent were large immature cells with large nuclei and basophilic cytoplasm. The bone marrow preparations showed total replacement by "blast" cells with inhibition of normal hematopoiesis in all three series. There were hyperuricemia and metabolic acidosis.

A diagnosis of congenital leukemia was made. Treatment with vincristine and steroids was started. An exchange transfusion was performed. The peripheral blood picture abated, but thrombocytopenia persisted and a generalized hemorrhagic syndrome appeared. Transfusions of whole blood and of concentrated platelets were performed. Two days before the child's demise blood culture was positive for *Candida* and diphtheroids. Death occurred on the twelfth day after birth.

Histopathologic Examination. The pancreatic acini are spread apart by a diffuse infiltration of leukemic cells (H & E, 375 ×).

Other findings: Bilateral necrotizing bronchopneumonia, septic foci in the liver, lymphoid depletion of lymph nodes, and atrophy of the thymus. No other areas of leukemic infiltration were found.

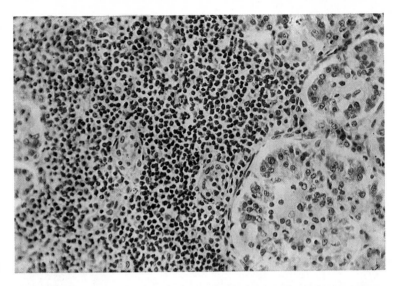

224

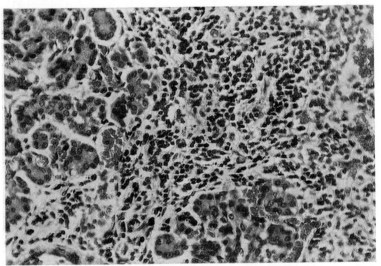

225

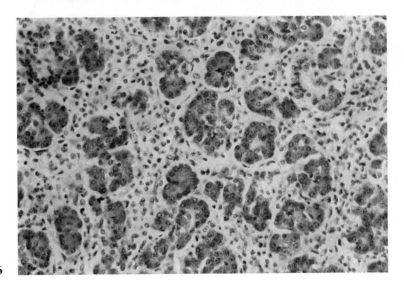

226

227/228
HYPERPLASIA OF ISLETS OF LANGERHANS

Female weighing 2,750 gm. Gestational age, 32 weeks. History is given with Figure 119.

Histopathologic Examination. Figure 227 shows a hyperplastic islet with a fibrous capsule vividly accentuated by this trichrome stain. In the center of the islet there is a cluster of hematopoietic cells (Masson, 187.5×).

Figure 228 shows infiltration by similar cells in the area surrounding an islet, with the participation of many eosinophils (H & E, 375 ×).

Hyperplasia of islets is found also in erythroblastosis and in some cases of spontaneous hypoglycemia. The low blood sugar level observed in infants with erythroblastosis could be related to this hyperplasia of islets.

Other findings: Pulmonary atelectasis of congestive type, with pulmonary hyaline membranes, cerebral and pulmonary petechiae, and moderate cardiomegaly (Fig. 119).

229
CYTOMEGALIC INCLUSION DISEASE INVOLVING PANCREATIC ISLETS

Female weighing 1,150 gm. Gestational age, 29 weeks. Admitted 2 hours after delivery with no other history. On admission, mild respiratory distress, hypotonia, obvious immaturity, and mixed acidosis were noted. The latter was treated with glucose-bicarbonate infusion. Beginning at 48 hours of life, respiratory insufficiency was complicated by grayish pallor, abdominal distention with some degree of superficial venous engorgement, general depression, and diarrheic stools. The general impression was that of sepsis. Blood culture was negative. Stool culture was positive for *E. coli* type 086B7, for which appropriate treatment was given. The intestinal picture improved, but hepatomegaly developed; symptoms of sepsis persisted, and marked jaundice became apparent. Total bilirubin was 10 mg/100 ml, direct 6.6 mg/100 ml, SGOT 725 U/L, and SGPT 372 U/L. The diagnosis of septic hepatitis was made. Another blood culture was negative and so was the search for cytomegalic inclusions in the urine. At 20 days of life there was renewed respiratory difficulty, and x-rays showed disseminated bronchopneumonic shadows. Mixed acidosis supervened, and the infant died at 22 days in respiratory arrest.

Histopathologic Examination. In one of the islets of Langerhans there is a large cell that shows within its nucleus a deeply basophilic inclusion with a clear halo around it; the chromatin is displaced toward the nuclear membrane (H & E, 600 ×).

Other findings: Disseminated bronchopneumonia and cytomegalic inclusion disease affecting a number of organs (Fig. 213).

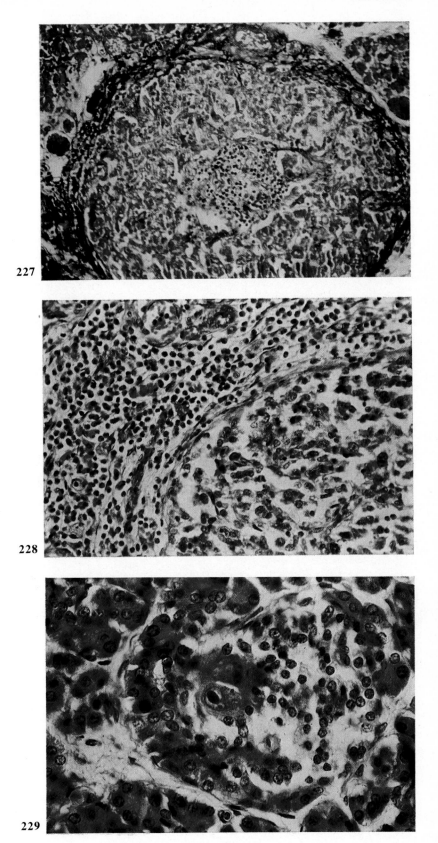

227

228

229

230
ABERRANT PANCREATIC TISSUE IN DUODENUM

Female weighing 2,000 gm. Gestational age, 34 weeks. Breech delivery. Apgar score 4. Intensive resuscitation was carried out. Admitted 1 hour later in serious respiratory difficulty. There was a 6 by 4 cm omphalocele. Crises of anoxia recurred, and the child died at 6 hours of age.

Histopathologic Examination. An island of pancreatic tissue can be seen in the wall of the duodenum. It lies partly in the submucosa and also dissects apart bundles of muscle in the muscularis propria (H & E, 60 ×). Pancreatic nodules are fairly common in the wall of the digestive tract from the pylorus to the terminal ileum.

Autopsy also showed an omphalocele unaccompanied by other anomalies. Other findings: Cerebral hemorrhage and petechiae on the pleural surfaces, pericardium, and thymus.

231
PANCREATICOSPLENIC FUSION

Female weighing 2,000 gm. Gestational age, 38 weeks. Apgar score 7 at 1 minute. Admitted at 3 hours of life in poor general condition with generalized cyanosis, low implantation of ears, broad nose, microophthalmia, unilateral harelip, cleft palate, midline defect of the scalp in the occipital region, anomalous placement of the toes, moderate respiratory distress, and signs of trisomy 13. Chest x-ray showed 11 ribs on each side, cardiomegaly, and atelectasis with mediastinal shift to the right.

She died 18 hours after admission. Karyotyping confirmed the diagnosis of trisomy 13.

Histopathologic Examination. The tail of the pancreas was inextricably attached to the spleen. Microscopically, both types of tissue were connected by a thin connective tissue band representing a common capsule, interrupted intermittently, that allowed direct contact and areas of fusion between the two parenchymas (H & E, 187.5 ×).

Other findings: Infratentorial hemorrhage and pulmonary atelectasis with some pulmonary hyaline membrane formation.

232
ECTOPIC PANCREATIC TISSUE IN SPLEEN

Male weighing 3,000 gm. Gestational age, 40 weeks. Breech delivery. Apgar score 5 at 1 minute after birth. Admitted at 1 hour of life, moribund, with severe respiratory distress, no spontaneous movements, microcephaly, odd-shaped ears implanted low, conspicuous microophthalmia, omphalocele, polydactyly, and a bean-sized patch of pink discoloration in the scalp.

Resuscitation with oxygen administration and bicarbonate acid glucose infusion. X-rays showed 11 ribs on either side, cardiomegaly, and situs inversus. Ophthalmologically, there was bilateral microophthalmia, coloboma, and fetal type of vitreous. Hematologically, there were nuclear abnormalities in 80 per cent of polymorphonuclear leukocytes; there were no Heinz bodies, and electrophoresis gave no evidence of Bart's hemoglobin. Cytogenetic studies on peripheral blood showed 47 chromosomes in all metaphase, with an accessory medium-sized element belonging to group D; the diagnosis of trisomy 13 was established.

Respiratory insufficiency progressed, and death occurred at 20 hours.

Histopathologic Examination. Nestled within splenic tissue there is a nodule of pancreatic tissue including acini and ducts with a fibrous stroma. There are no changes in the splenic tissue itself (H & E, 187.5 ×).

Autopsy showed the features of trisomy 13 with situs inversus and arrhinencephaly. There was massive pulmonary hemorrhage.

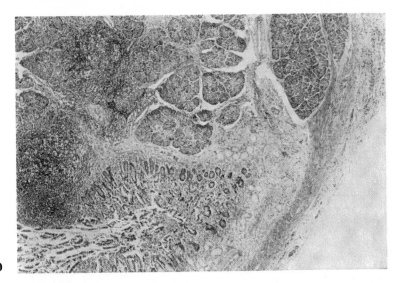

230

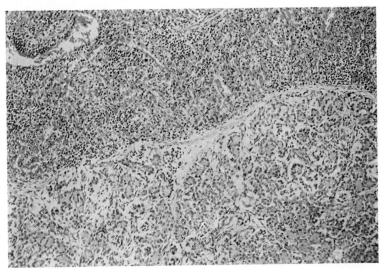

231

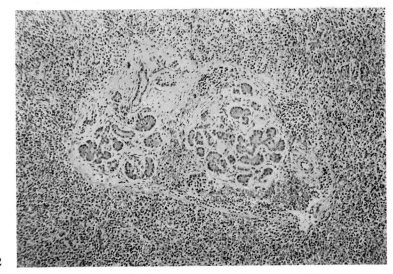

232

233
ANOXIC NECROSIS OF ISLETS OF LANGERHANS

Male weighing 3,040 gm. Gestational age, 36 weeks. Rupture of membranes 10 hours before delivery. Precipitous delivery. Admitted 2 hours later with weak cry, generalized cyanosis, hypotonia, hypothermia, shallow breathing, expiratory grunt, hyporeflexia, and severe metabolic acidosis. Bicarbonate infusion by umbilical route induced slight improvement, but multiple bouts of apnea followed, and in one of them the infant died 8 hours after birth.

Histopathologic Examination. The architecture of the exocrine pancreas is intact. On the other hand, islets of Langerhans such as the one in Figure 233 are necrotic; the nuclei of most of the cells have lost their detail (H & E, 375 ×).

Other findings: Signs of anoxia in various organs, renal tubular necrosis, and multiple hemorrhagic foci in viscera, especially in the lung.

234
FOCAL PANCREATIC MICRODYSPLASIA

Female weighing 1,840 gm. Unknown gestational age. Admitted at 3 days of life.

On admission she gave the impression of suffering from sepsis. General condition was poor; she was deeply jaundiced, had moderate respiratory distress and gastrointestinal upset. Blood and urine cultures were negative, but stool cultures produced colonies of *Staphylococcus* and *Candida*.

Plain film of the abdomen showed air shadows limited to the proximal portions of the small bowel. Twenty-four hours after admission the respiratory deficit increased and bloody secretions oozed from the upper airway. This was followed by abdominal distention and fatal collapse.

Histopathologic Examination. Most of the samples of pancreatic tissue examined appeared normal. In one section, however, there was a small area that exhibited atrophy, sclerosis, and cystic transformation of acini and ducts. Note the normal structure of adjacent pancreatic tissue (H & E, 60 ×).

Other findings: Purulent peritonitis due to perforation of the bowel, advanced enteritis, and focal pulmonary hemorrhages (Fig. 218).

235
FOCAL CYSTIC DYSPLASIA OF PANCREAS

Eighteen day old infant weighing 3,650 gm. Admitted for diarrhea, dehydration, and poor general condition. pH 7.17, pCO_2 32.5 mm Hg, BE − 16 mEq/L, chloride 109 mEq/L, sodium 141 mEq/L, potassium 4.2 mEq/L, microhematocrit 28 per cent. Stool culture yielded enteropathogenic *E. coli*, type 0:111–B4, and *Candida*.

Rehydration and correction of acidosis were begun. Respiratory difficulty was manifest, and chest films showed bilateral confluent infiltrates. There was no response to treatment, and the child died in 48 hours.

Histopathologic Examination. At one end of the section there is a group of ducts showing large, cystic lumina, each lined by a single layer of epithelium. The remainder of the parenchyma shows no changes (H & E, 60 ×).

Other findings: Monocytic bronchopneumonia with a marked hemorrhagic component, severe enteritis.

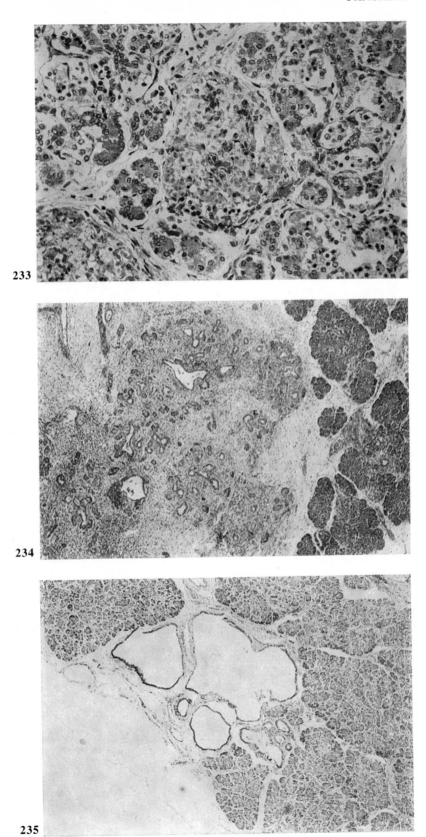

233

234

235

236

CYSTIC FIBROSIS OF PANCREAS

Female weighing 3,900 gm. Gestational age, 40 weeks. Admitted at 24 hours of age because of abdominal distention and failure to pass meconium (history is given with Figures 94 and 95).

Histopathologic Examination. The pancreas shows marked increase of connective tissue, which forms bands among the glandular acini. The latter are dilated. In some areas microcystic structures can be seen, filled with dense mucinous material.

Other findings: Extensive pulmonary changes (Figs. 94 and 95) and purulent peritonitis.

237

ADVANCED CYSTIC FIBROSIS OF PANCREAS

Twenty-eight day old infant weighing 3,600 gm. From the time of birth he had passed very fetid diarrheic stools. Simultaneously he exhibited a respiratory picture reminiscent of whooping cough. On admission he had dyspnea, cyanosis, nasal flutter, and fever. Chest films showed marked homogeneous emphysema with widening of intercostal spaces and low diaphragm. Both parahilar regions showed nodularity and small trabecular opacities suggesting atelectasis. At both bases, around and behind the cardiac shadows there were coarse bronchial "broom-like" markings. The cardiovascular outlines seemed normal, though somewhat encroached upon by emphysema.

Sweat electrolyte level was 85 mEq/L. Biopsy of the lip did not show any cystic dilatation of glands.

With a working diagnosis of mucoviscidosis, treatment was instituted. The respiratory component did not improve. One month after admission the child died in respiratory failure.

Histopathologic Examination. For the most part, pancreatic parenchyma is replaced by hyalinized fibrous tissue. Within it are seen islets of Langerhans and remnants of exocrine pancreas including cystically dilated ducts (Masson, 187.5 ×).

The autopsy findings were those of typical cystic fibrosis of the pancreas with disseminated bronchopneumonia.

238

DUODENUM IN CYSTIC FIBROSIS OF PANCREAS

Twenty-five day old male weighing 3,550 gm. Admitted for an acute respiratory process. There was a history of delay in evacuation of meconium and 6 days of respiratory difficulty consisting of intercostal retraction and expiratory grunting. Chest x-ray showed signs of atelectasis and emphysema by confluent nodular shadows consistent with bronchopneumonia. Repeated bouts of apnea required resuscitation. Stools had been normal up to that point. A sample of sweat showed 97 mEq/L of sodium chloride.

Mixed metabolic and respiratory acidosis and multiple respiratory arrests eventuated in death 3 days after admission.

Histopathologic Examination. Figure 238 shows a section of duodenal wall. Dilatation of Brunner's glands is quite obvious (H & E, 375×).

Other findings: Changes typical of cystic fibrosis of the pancreas and bilateral diffuse bronchopneumonia.

239

GALLBLADDER IN CYSTIC FIBROSIS OF THE PANCREAS

For history see text for Figures 94, 95, and 236.

Histopathologic Examination. Figure 239 shows marked dilatation of the glands of the neck of the gallbladder, which are filled with PAS-positive mucinous material (PAS, 375 ×).

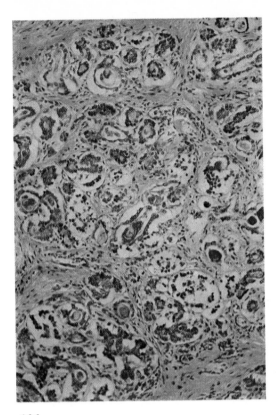

236

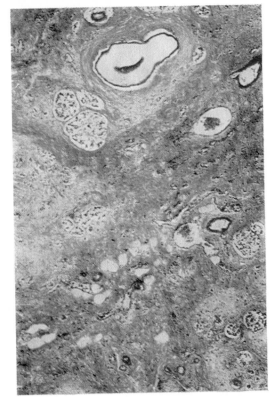

237

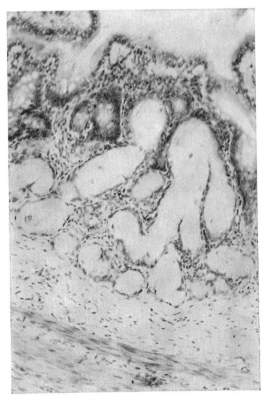

238

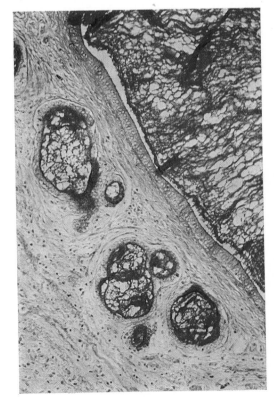

239

Liver

240/241
HEPATIC IMMATURITY

Male weighing 1,000 gm. Gestational age, 27 weeks. Vertex delivery. Rupture of membranes 5 days before. Apgar score 3 at 3 minutes.

On admission, poor general condition, generalized cyanosis, hypotonia, gasping respirations, and metabolic acidosis.

The infant was placed in an incubator under standard conditions and given 10 per cent glucose and 1 M bicarbonate infusion. He died 2 hours later.

Histopathologic Examinations. The portal space shown in Figure 240 is widened, apparently by fibrosis. Within it there are immature blood cells and eosinophils. Comparable hematopoietic activity can be observed in the sinusoids of the liver (H & E, 187.5 ×).

Figure 241 demonstrates in greater detail an increase in the thickness of liver trabeculae. The sinusoids are dilated and filled with blood containing hematopoietic elements (H & E, 375×).

242
ABNORMAL PERSISTENCE OF HEMATOPOIETIC ACTIVITY

Twenty-day old male weighing 2,610 gm. Reason for admission: Frequent vomiting, unrelated to feedings and without bile staining, since the day of birth, accompanied by constipation.

Physical examination immediately disclosed Down's syndrome and congenital cardiac disease. The latter was identified as a high interventricular septal defect with hypoplasia of the left chambers. Metabolic alkalosis was recognized and corrected.

Radiographic studies demonstrated duodenal stenosis, possibly related to annular pancreas. Surgery corroborated that diagnosis. Repair was carried out, and the child was discharged in satisfactory condition 12 days later. He was readmitted after 10 days with heart failure. Despite digitalization he survived only a week.

Histopathologic Examinations. The architecture of the liver is normal. The presence of small foci of hematopoietic activity is an unexpected feature in view of the patient's age (H & E, 375 ×). Similar nests were found in the spleen. The explanation for this persistence of extramedullary hematopoietic activity probably lies in the presence of sustained anoxia.

Other findings: High, large interventricular septal defect, hypoplasia of left side of the heart and hypertrophy of the right ventricle.

243
EOSINOPHILIC LEUKEMIA (?)

Male weighing 3,500 gm, admitted at 22 days of age. On examination the infant showed typical Down's syndrome. There were erythematous areas on the face, lower extremities, and trunk. There were no indurated or nodular skin lesions. A very large spleen was palpable.

Hematologic studies: Microhematocrit 51 per cent, wbc 82,000, basophils 4 per cent, myelocytes 2 per cent, metamyelocytes 1 per cent, segmented 9 per cent, lymphocytes 5 per cent, monocytes 2 per cent, blast forms 46 per cent, eosinophils 31 per cent (9 per cent myelocytic and promyelocytic, 5 per cent metamyelocytic, 5 per cent band forms, and 12 per cent segmented); platelets 60,000/cu mm.

The bone marrow showed: Erythroblasts 3.5 per cent, myelocytes 0.5 per cent, metamyelocytes 3.5 per cent, blast forms 26 per cent. The eosinophils were present in all stages of maturation. Many of them, especially in the early stages, showed clearly atypical features and contained fat-positive granules. The blast forms were reminiscent of paramyeloblasts and were negative for fat and peroxidase stains. There was general PAS positivity of eosinophils, while blasts were PAS-negative.

Total protein 4.8 gm/100 ml; albumin 3.8 gm/100 ml; alpha 1 globulin 0.23, alpha 2 globulin 0.29, beta globulin 0.29, and gamma globulin 0.19 mg/100 ml. Urine culture was positive for *E. coli* (3,200,000 colonies per milliliter). A liver biopsy was done.

Initially a diagnosis of eosinophilic leukemia was made, and chemotherapeutic treatment was instituted. A complete remission was obtained as indicated by blood and bone marrow studies, and the child was discharged 1 month later. The final diagnosis was held in abeyance because of the complete disappearance of the clinical symptoms (save for the persistence of a slight hepatosplenomegaly) and the sustained normality of blood studies for 5 months.

Histopathologic Examination. The trabecular pattern of the lobules is distorted by infiltration of immature cells. Eosinophils predominate, some of them segmented (H & E, 375×). Similar but less pronounced infiltration appeared in the portal spaces. Compare this type of infiltration with that illustrated in Figure 240.

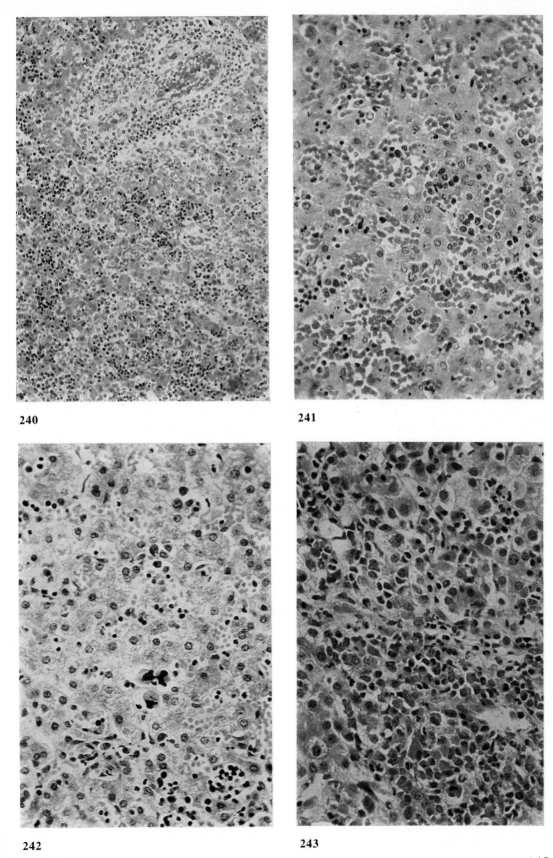

240

241

242

243

244

PASSIVE CONGESTION OF THE LIVER

Female weighing 2,150 gm. Unknown gestational age. Rupture of membranes 7 days prior to a rather stormy delivery. Admitted at 2 hours of life in poor general condition with moderate hypotonia, depressed motor activity, and inadequate sucking reflex. Some degree of generalized edema was present. There was no passage of meconium until the fourth day. Jaundice appeared on the third day, and 24 hours later the level of the total bilirubin was 17.5 per cent. White blood cells numbered 8,500/cu mm with a marked shift to the left. General condition remained unsatisfactory, and a grayish pallor developed. There was no increase in weight. Jaundice persisted. Ulcerated lesions appeared in the upper maxillary area and in the vulva. Severe metabolic acidosis developed. Clinically she had sepsis. There was no response to treatment, and death occurred at 20 days.

Histopathologic Examination. The liver weighed 118 gm. The cut surface showed the characteristic "nutmeg" pattern. Figure 244 illustrates marked dilatation of the liver sinusoids, which are engorged with blood, and partial flattening of the trabeculae (H & E, 375 ×).

The final diagnosis: Sepsis with bilateral extensive areas of hemorrhagic pneumonia and mucocutaneous necrotizing hemorrhagic lesions.

245

PORTAL THROMBOSIS AND FOCAL HEPATIC NECROSIS

Male weighing 3,300 gm. Gestational age, 40 weeks. Vertex delivery 7 hours after rupture of membranes. On admission, examination revealed anal atresia, laryngeal stridor, hypospadias, and moderate respiratory insufficiency.

Chest x-rays showed right apical cloudiness, probably related to aspiration. A nasogastric tube passed readily into the stomach, excluding the possibility of esophageal atresia. Bicarbonate perfusion corrected the existing moderate acidosis. Culture of gastric contents yielded *Klebsiella pneumoniae.*

Two days later the anal atresia was corrected surgically. On resumption of oral feedings, suspicion of tracheoesophageal fistula arose. Intravenous alimentation was restarted. Signs of respiratory insufficiency appeared. Chest films showed bilateral bronchopneumonia.

Recurring bouts of respiratory arrest were treated but the infant died at 10 days of life.

Histopathologic Examination. There was thrombosis of the left branch of the portal vein. An extensive portion of the left lobe of the liver showed hemorrhagic infarction. Figure 245 represents the area of necrosis as contrasted with normal liver tissue occupying the right lower portion of the field. In the portal space, in the center, the bile canaliculi appear well preserved, but the interlobular portal branches are thrombosed (H & E, 60 ×).

Other findings: Rectourethral fistula, hypospadias, and high tracheoesophageal fistula.

246

SUBCAPSULAR HEMATOMA OF THE LIVER

Male weighing 3,760 gm. Gestational age, 40 weeks. Vertex delivery after 1 hour of labor. Apgar score 9 at birth. A few hours later the child appeared generally ill, with depressed sensorium, marked pallor of skin and mucosae, vascular collapse, weak cry, shallow respirations, tachypnea, hypotonia, hyporeflexia, apical systolic murmur, and 4 cm hepatomegaly. Studies: Microhematocrit 18 per cent, pH 6.72, BE −22 mEq/L. Films of the abdomen were made. A diagnosis of hemoperitoneum—the result of laceration of the liver—was suggested. A transfusion was given. An hour later the hematocrit was 19 per cent, pH 7.05, BE −18 mEq/L. Infusion of dextrose-bicarbonate solution, which had been started, was continued. Laparotomy disclosed abundant intraperitoneal blood, which was traced to a 3 cm tear in the capsule of the right lobe of the liver. The lesion was repaired.

Coagulation tests prior to transfusion had shown deficient clotting. After surgery a 100 ml transfusion was performed, consisting of blood and 1 M bicarbonate solution. Three hours later the pH was 7.36 and BE −5 mEq/L. Shortly thereafter considerable bleeding occurred. Suddenly minor convulsions appeared and breathing became difficult. Cardiorespiratory arrest followed and could not be reversed.

Histopathologic Examination. Figure 246 shows the appearance of the subcapsular hepatic hematoma with a wide-meshed fibrin network in the interstices of which are many red cells, visible in the upper right portion of the figure (H & E, 187.5×).

Autopsy also revealed an extensive subarachnoid hemorrhage, and hemorrhagic lesions in adrenals, kidneys, and lungs.

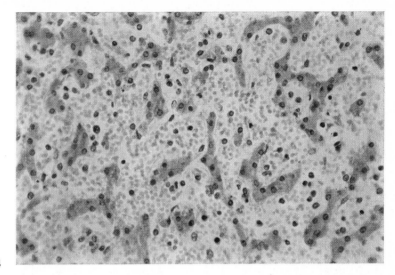

244

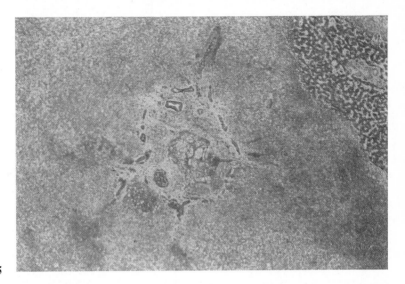

245

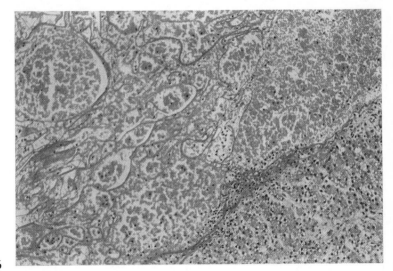

246

247/248
ERYTHROBLASTOSIS

Male weighing 2,400 gm. Unknown gestational age. Admitted at 2 hours of life in poor condition with hypotonia, hypothermia, decreased motor activity, edema, moderate dyspnea, jaundice, pallor, and hepatosplenomegaly. Blood type: A, Rh positive (D). The mother was Rh negative. Positive direct Coombs test. At 3 hours, hematocrit 31 per cent, total bilirubin 7.2 mg/100 ml, total protein 4.6 gm/100 ml, pH 7.11, pCO_2 45 mm Hg., BE -16.5 mEq/L. An intravenous infusion of bicarbonate in dextrose solution was given. At 7 hours there was no improvement. Total bilirubin 14.4 mg/100 ml, microhematocrit 29 per cent, total protein 3.6 gm/100 ml, pH 7.26, pCO_2 65 mm Hg, BE -3 mEq/L. Again 1 M bicarbonate was administered, and an exchange transfusion was carried out by the umbilical route, using 400 ml of A Rh negative packed red blood cells.

In the next few hours the infant improved. The following day, however, his condition deteriorated. Total bilirubin, 17.28 mg/100 ml. Another exchange transfusion was done. After that the bilirubin went to 5.8 mg/100 ml and the infant improved, only to develop respiratory distress and to expel bloody mucus by mouth. Recurrent bouts of apnea required repeated resuscitative maneuvers. The bilirubin 8 hours after the preceding determination was 22.4 mg/100 ml total and 6.6 mg/100 ml direct. The patient's condition at that time appeared terminal, and he required assisted respiration. Death occurred 2 hours later.

Histopathologic Examination. Figure 247 shows hematopoietic foci between liver trabeculae. The erythroblastic series predominate (H & E, 600 ×). This activity is out of proportion to the degree of maturity of the liver. Within hepatocytes, a brown granular pigment appears that takes on a blue color with Prussian blue stain (Fig. 248, 600 ×).

Other findings: There were substantial foci of hematopoiesis in the spleen and adrenals. The basal ganglia of the brain showed marked bile staining. There was massive pulmonary hemorrhage and moderate aspiration of meconium.

249/250
CONGENITAL FIBROCYSTIC DYSPLASIA

Female weighing 2,380 gm. Gestational age, 30 weeks. Born by breech delivery. Apgar score 4 at 1 minute. Admitted 2 hours later in poor condition, with cyanosis and serious respiratory difficulty. Chest x-rays showed inadequate expansion, especially on the right. There was a fracture of the right femur. The skin bore scattered petechiae. A large mass occupied the entire abdomen. Its outlines were vague, but it seemed to represent enlarged kidneys. Studies: pH 6.9 pCO_2 100 mm Hg, BE -12 mEq/L. Bicarbonate-dextrose solution was administered by the umbilical route.

One hour after admission respiratory arrest occurred, necessitating intubation and assisted respiration. Three hours later the child died.

Histopathologic Examination. The liver was normal in size and its surface was smooth. On the cut surface the portal areas were quite visible, pale and arborescent. The gallbladder was hypoplastic, but the bile ducts were patent.

Microscopically, with Masson's trichrome stain the variable size of the portal spaces is accentuated. All of them show fibrosis. The bile canaliculi are large and branching. Vessels are scarce in the portal areas; in this illustration only one blood space, above and to the center, stands out (Fig. 249, 60 ×). With greater magnification, the tortuous configuration of the bile ducts can be seen. The lining of each consists of normal cylindrical cells. The large cystic cavity shows a number of fibroepithelial villous formations projecting into the lumen. There is no inflammatory infiltration of the portal spaces (Fig. 250, 375 ×). In older children, signs of cholangitis are a frequent accompaniment.

Other findings: There were abundant hematopoietic elements in the parenchymal sinusoids. The kidneys showed infantile polycystic transformation. The lungs were hypoplastic (22 gm in contrast to a normal 49 gm) and contained interstitial hemorrhages. There were anoxic petechiae in the brain, trachea, and digestive tract. The heart showed marked fibrosis of papillary muscles.

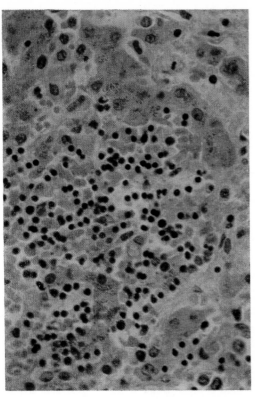

247

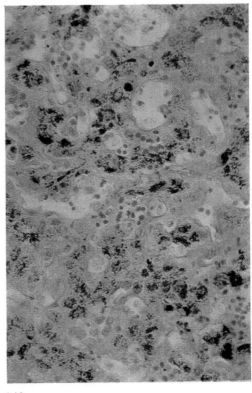

248

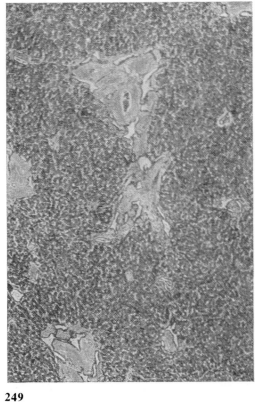

249

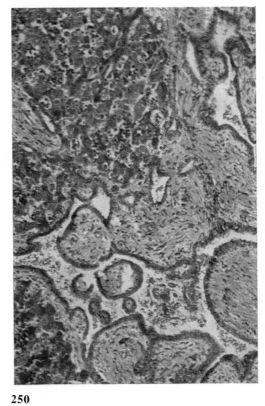

250

251/252
ATRESIA OF EXTRAHEPATIC BILE DUCTS

Twenty-five day old male born at term weighing 3,100 gm. Admitted for progressive jaundice with acholia and choluria, moderate hypotonia, fever, and restlessness for 2 days.

Examination revealed intense jaundice of the skin and mucosal surfaces, abdominal distention with some collateral circulation, and palpable liver 3 fingerbreadths below the costal margin; no splenomegaly. Total bilirubin 9.06 mg/100 ml, SGOT 185 u/L, SGPT 300 u/L, microhematocrit 31 per cent, Hb 9.8 gm/100 ml, rose bengal-I[131] Nordyke test 77.5 per cent and 4.58 per cent fecal excretion of tracer dose in 72 hours.

Surgical exploration showed the distal biliary pathways to be patent. There was no sign of passage of contrast medium back into the liver, however. A diagnosis of radicular type of extrahepatic bile duct atresia was made.

Histopathologic Examination. The material examined represents a surgical liver biopsy. The most conspicuous observations in Figure 251 are fibrosis of portal areas, which tends to be confluent, and proliferation of the bile ducts (Masson, 187.5 ×).

Portal spaces show deposits of immunoglobulin G in the connective tissue (fluorescence with fluoresceine isothiocyanate-labeled anti-IgG antiglobulin) (Masson, 187.5 ×).

Comment: On occasion, the differential diagnosis in biopsy material between atresia of extrahepatic bile ducts and neonatal hepatitis is difficult. One of the significant signs of atresia is the proliferation of bile canaliculi in the portal areas, frequently accompanied by hypertrophy of the muscular coat of the interlobular branch of the hepatic artery. The presence of bile pigment within the portal bile ducts is not a constant finding. (Translators' note: In our experience it is often positive and an indication of atresia.) As for bile plugs within the lobule, it must be recalled that cholestasis may be observed in the so-called dense bile syndrome in erythroblastosis, in which bile capillaries are dilated and filled with bile. Portal infiltration is usually a restrained component in extrahepatic atresia. In extrahepatic obstruction, as by a choledochal cyst, polymorphonuclear leukocytes may be found in portal spaces. In neonatal hepatitis round cell portal infiltration is a prominent feature and there are hepatocellular changes. It should be pointed out that the classic concept of the congenital nature of biliary atresia is hardly tenable at present. Both atresia and neonatal hepatitis are probably related to an inflammatory process that may have two different modalities of morphologic expression or development. Both may be manifestations of the same basic disease.

253/254
ATRESIA OF EXTRAHEPATIC BILE DUCTS

Twenty-eight day old male. Gestational age, 37 weeks. Weight at birth 2,100 gm. The immediate neonatal period was normal. The family history included a sibling afflicted with atresia of extrahepatic bile ducts who died of cirrhosis at 2 years of age.

This child was admitted because of jaundice of 10 days' duration, choluria, increasing acholia, and 2 fingerbreadth hepatomegaly without a palpable spleen. Studies: Microhematocrit 37 per cent, Hb 12 gm/100 ml, bilirubin total 7.9 mg/100 ml, direct 6.9 mg/100 ml, SGOT 106 u/L, SGPT 94 u/L, LDH 73 u/L, alkaline phosphatase 6.8 Bodansky units; total lipids 662 mg/100 ml, total protein 6.2 gm/100 ml, albumin 51.9 per cent, rose bengal−I[131] Nordyke test 80.9 per cent, 72 hour fecal excretion of tracer 2.2 per cent.

Exploratory laparotomy exposed a dark, firm liver. Cholangiography resulted in visualization of an atrophic gallbladder. There was no passage of contrast medium to extrahepatic bile ducts. A surgical liver biopsy was performed.

Histopathologic Examination. Figure 253 shows marked portal fibrosis with scanty cellularity. There is perceptible hyperplasia of an interlobular branch of the hepatic artery (Masson, 600 ×).

This vascular change, although not specific, is frequently observed in atresia of extrahepatic bile ducts, including that seen in stillborn infants. (Translators' note: We have not yet observed extrahepatic biliary atresia in a stillborn infant.)

Figure 254 shows cholestasis in the central portions of lobules, characterized by large, dense bile thrombi in bile capillaries (H & E, 600 ×).

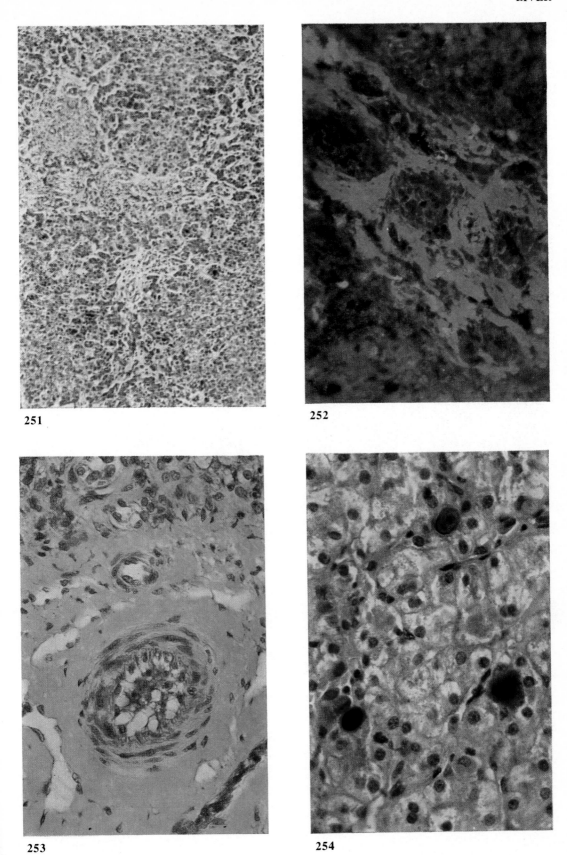

251

252

253

254

255/256
CONGENITAL CYST OF COMMON DUCT

Twenty-five day old male, born at term, weighing 3,700 gm. Admitted with mild jaundice, poor general condition, respiratory difficulty, whining, weak cry, hypothermia, bulging fontanelle under tension, myoclonus in upper extremities, vertical nystagmus, and 2 finger-breadth hepatomegaly.

Studies: Total bilirubin 5.7 mg/100 ml, direct 4.9 mg/100 ml, microhematocrit 20 per cent, SGOT 90 u/L, SGPT 100 u/L. EEG was abnormal with decreased activity. Spinal tap released hemorrhagic fluid, negative on culture. Blood and urine cultures were negative. Chest films showed disseminated bronchopneumonia. There was mixed respiratory and metabolic acidosis. Coagulation time was more than 1 hour and was not improved by the addition of calcium or thromboplastin. The addition of thrombin brought it to normal.

Diagnosis: Subarachnoid hemorrhage related to a coagulopathy caused by liver disease with complicating bronchopneumonia. The infant died 48 hours after admission.

Histopathologic Examination. The liver was normal in size. Its surface was finely irregular. It cut with increased resistance, and the cut surface was greenish-brown. The gallbladder was normal and contained clear mucus. The cystic duct was dilated and opened into a cystically transformed common duct. Postmortem injection of dye demonstrated the failure of passage of contrast medium into the duodenum, whereas there was good communication between hepatic ducts and the gallbladder.

Histopathologic study shows increased connective tissue and marked bile duct proliferation in the portal spaces (Fig. 255, H & E, 375×). Figure 256 shows higher magnification of an enlarged portal space. Note the hyperplasia of the interlobular arterial branch and its caliber, which is greater than that of the bile ducts.

The clinical diagnoses of intracranial hemorrhage and bronchopneumonia were confirmed as the causes of the infant's death.

257
ATRESIA OF EXTRAHEPATIC BILE DUCTS

Twenty-five day old male born at term weighing 3,630 gm, admitted with a history of jaundice since the fourth day of life. Jaundice had increased progressively and was accompanied by choluria and acholia.

On admission the infant's general condition was satisfactory; jaundice was obvious, and the stool was acholic. Studies: Total bilirubin 20.5 mg/100 ml, direct 15 mg/100 ml, microhematocrit 26 per cent, total protein 5.0 gm/100 ml, SGOT 450 u/L, SGPT 680 u/l, cholesterol 295 mg/100 ml, prothrombin time 18 seconds. The rose bengal–I^{131} test showed 4.6 per cent fecal excretion of the tracer in 72 hours. Exploratory laparotomy revealed absence of extrahepatic biliary tract. The operative cholangiogram showed a noncommunicating gallbladder. A surgical liver biopsy was done. Postoperative follow-up led to the final diagnosis of cirrhosis.

Histopathologic Examination. The biopsy showed the picture of bile duct atresia. The presence of multinucleated giant cells containing bile pigment in their cytoplasm is to be noted (H & E, 600 ×). Giant cells are seen occasionally in instances of atresia of the extrahepatic bile ducts. They are in no way specific for so-called neonatal giant cell hepatitis.

258
ATRESIA OF EXTRAHEPATIC BILE DUCTS

Twenty-day old female born at term with a weight of 3,700 gm. At 3 days of life the infant developed jaundice, which increased and was accompanied by choluria and acholia. Admitted for study. On admission there were frank jaundice and acholia but good general condition. Total bilirubin 15.22 mg/100 ml, direct 13.8 mg/100 ml, microhematocrit 29 per cent, SGOT 310 u/L, SGPT 360 u/L, cholesterol 255 mg/100 ml, alkaline phosphatase 14 Bodansky units, gamma globulin 3.5 mg/100 ml, I^{131}–rose bengal test results: Nordyke test 82.7 per cent 72 hour excretion 4.3 per cent.

Exploratory laparotomy demonstrated absence of extrahepatic bile ducts and rudimentary gallbladder. Biliary tree was replaced by fibrous tracts. Liver biopsy was done.

Histopathologic Examination. Figure 258 shows intralobular bile canaliculi stained by the ATP-ase method. There are short, irregular segments with marked ampullary dilatations in the center. The contours of the sinusoids show increased enzymatic activity (375×).

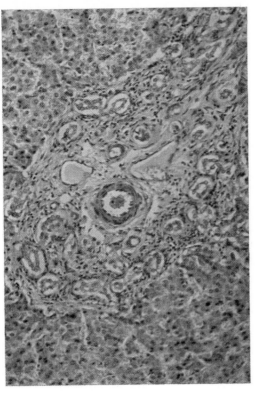

255

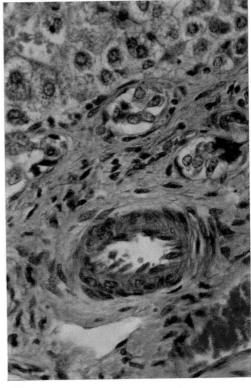

256

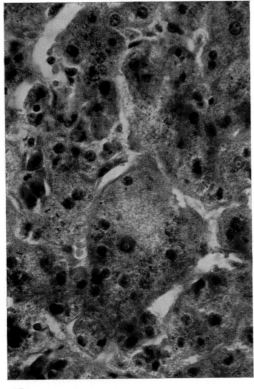

257

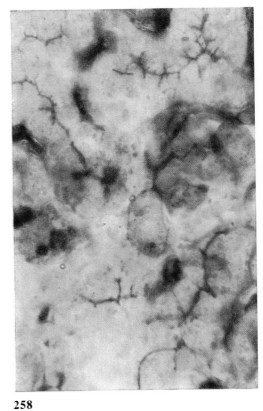

258

ATRESIA OF EXTRAHEPATIC BILE DUCTS

Same patient as in Figure 258.

Histopathologic Examination. In the biopsy fragment studied for leucilaminopeptidase activity the interlobular canaliculi and the bile capillaries are selectively outlined. Figure 259 shows proliferation of bile ducts in the portal areas and perfectly regular intralobular capillary network. The brown centrolobular accumulations correspond to unstained bile pigment (187.5 ×).

The diaphorase method (NADH-tetrazolium reductase) stains all cytoplasm evenly except for the cells that line the bile-filled, dilated bile canaliculi (Fig. 260, succinohydrogenase, 600×).

EXTRAHEPATIC BILE DUCT ATRESIA

Twenty-five day old female born at term with a weight of 4,250 gm. Admitted because of jaundice dating from the first few days of life. For 5 days before admission she had exhibited acholia and marked choluria.

On admission her general condition was good, but there was deep jaundice. The spleen was palpable, and the liver was palpable 3 fingerbreadths below the costal margin. Total bilirubin 7.2 mg/100 ml, direct 6.4 mg/100 ml, cholesterol 207 mg/100 ml, SGOT 61 u/L, SGPT 120 u/L, LDH 58 u/L, aldolase 8.5 u/ml, alkaline phosphatase 8.3 Bodansky units. I^{131}—rose bengal test showed 75.8 per cent on Nordyke test and 2.67 per cent fecal excretion in 72 hours.

Exploratory laparotomy revealed total atresia of the extrahepatic bile ducts. A liver biopsy was performed.

Histopathologic Examination. Acid phosphatase stain for the lysosomic component of the cytoplasm showed marked activity in the liver cells surrounding the bile thrombi (Fig. 261, 600 ×).

Dilatation of the intralobular bile canaliculi is very conspicuous in Figure 262, the section stained for 5-nucleotidase. Next to some normal bile capillaries, others are seen that exhibit marked saccular transformation and increased enzymatic activity around bile thrombi (600 ×).

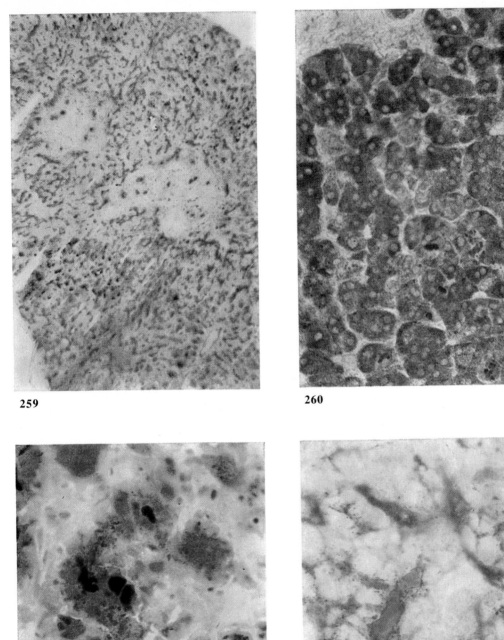

259

260

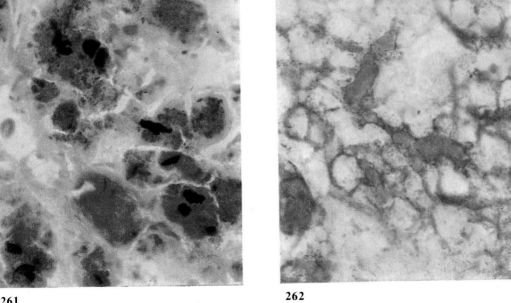

261

262

263/264/265/266
EXTRAHEPATIC BILE DUCT ATRESIA. CIRRHOSIS OF THE LIVER

Twenty-day old female, born at term, weighing 3,850 gm. Admitted for persistent jaundice since early life.

Examination showed intense jaundice, choluria, moderate acholia, and cutaneous petechiae as well as hepatomegaly, 2 fingerbreadths below the costal margin.

Total bilirubin 8.18 mg/100 ml, direct 5.9 mg/100 ml, SGOT 140 u/L, SGPT 176 u/L, cholesterol 299 mg/100 ml, I^{131}–rose bengal test resulted in 2.79 per cent excretion in 72 hours.

Laparotomy with operative cholangiogram demonstrated patency of the distal portion of the biliary tree with passage of contrast medium into the duodenum and atresia of the hepatic ducts impeding reflux of the medium into the liver.

In succeeding months there were several admissions for intercurrent infections and an episode of interstitial pneumonitis. A second biopsy was done when the patient was 19 months old.

Histopathologic Examination. Figure 263 shows marked fibrosis of the liver that has effaced the normal architecture. The parenchyma is reduced to two islands in this field (Masson, 60 ×).

Diaphorase stain shows persistence of enzyme activity in the residual islands. Nearby, there are many bile ducts (Fig. 264, 60 ×).

In Figure 265, an alkaline phosphatase stain reveals marked enzyme activity in the periphery of the residual liver parenchyma (60 ×). Acid phosphatase activity is much increased within the residual nodules, particularly in the vicinity of cholestatic foci (Fig. 266, 60 ×).

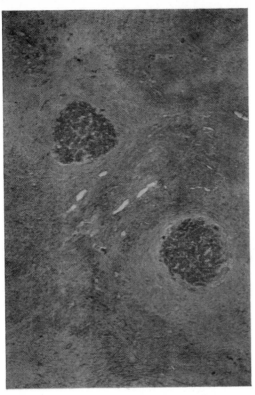

263

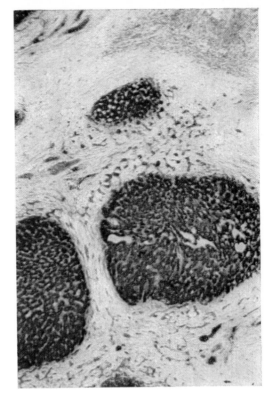

264

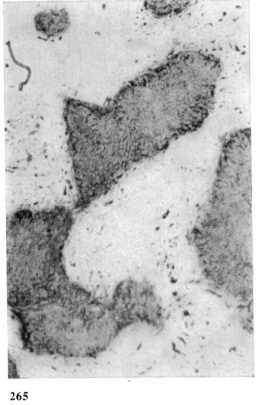

265

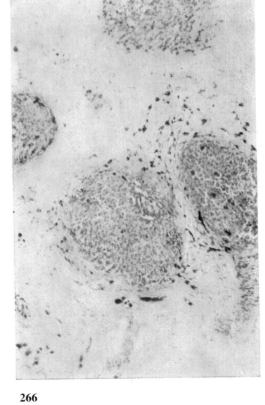

266

267/268/269
ATRESIA OF INTRAHEPATIC BILE DUCTS

Female weighing 2,840 gm, of unknown gestational age. Admitted at 18 days of life because of persistent jaundice from early life, choluria, and repeated vomiting.

Poor general condition, pale feces without frank acholia, deep jaundice, 1 fingerbreadth hepatomegaly, and metabolic acidosis. Total bilirubin 9.3 mg/100 ml, direct 6.08 mg/100 ml, SGOT 290 u/L, SGPT 320 u/L.

Negative blood and urine cultures. Acidosis was corrected, and the infant's general condition improved, but her jaundice deepened, taking on a greenish hue. I^{131}–rose bengal test gave an 83 per cent Nordyke result, and fecal excretion in 72 hours was 6.32 per cent. Malformation of the biliary tract was suspected, and a liver biopsy was done. The infant's condition deteriorated, and she died at 2 months of age.

Histopathologic Examination. Figure 267 shows a large portal area with no bile canaliculi. Note the presence of centrolobular bile stasis (H & E, 375 ×).

In Figure 268 changes in the normal reticulin network of the lobule can be observed. The normal trabecular arrangement is replaced by one that is pseudoacinar. In the center, there is a markedly dilated bile canaliculus containing a bile thrombus (Wilder, 600 ×).

Figure 269 shows the structure of a sample of liver taken at autopsy. A leucil-aminopeptidase stain selectively brings out the biliary network. Enzyme activity is obvious at the level of the intralobular bile capillaries, but it is lacking in the portal area because of the absence of bile ducts (187.5 ×). Compare this picture with that of extrahepatic biliary duct atresia seen in Figure 259.

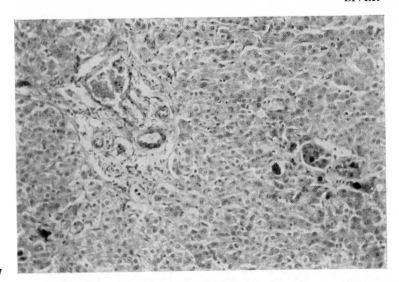

267

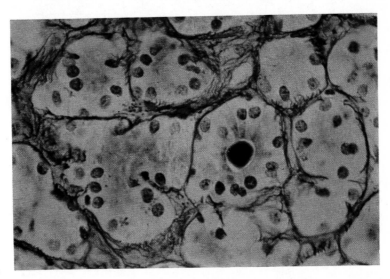

268

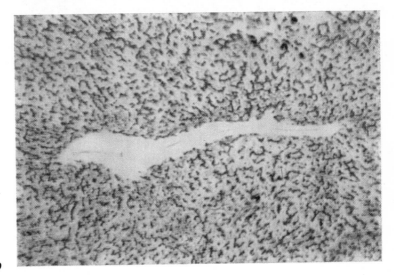

269

NEONATAL GIANT CELL HEPATITIS

Female weighing 1,150 gm, of 32 weeks' gestational age, twin birth, vertex delivery. Rupture of membranes moments before delivery. Admitted at 3 days of age with sclerema and jaundice. Total bilirubin 18.6 mg/100 ml. Metabolic acidosis, corrected by dextrose-bicarbonate solution.

In the next few days the bilirubin values dropped, suggesting a favorable outcome. On the fifteenth day of life, however, jaundice began to increase again. The infant's general condition deteriorated; the liver became palpable to 2 fingerbreadths. The baby was kept in an incubator. Total bilirubin 9.7 mg/100 ml, direct 8.3 mg/100 ml, SGOT 550 u/L, SGPT 440 u/L.

In the next few days the patient's general condition remained poor; bouts of metabolic acidosis were treated with bicarbonate solution. Culture of feces yielded colonies of *Aerobacter*. Blood and urine cultures were negative. There were no cytomegalic cells in the urine.

At 28 days of life jaundice continued; the feces were colored. Total bilirubin 11.8 mg/100 ml, direct 11.3 mg/100 ml, SGOT 612 u/L, SGPT 600 u/L. A diagnosis of neonatal hepatitis was made. Poor general condition continued, with jaundice and acidosis, until the fiftieth day, when the infant died.

Histopathologic Examination. The hepatic architecture is severely distorted, and transformation of hepatocytes into syncytial multinucleated cells containing bile granules is a prominent feature. Round cell infiltration in the interstitial spaces is conspicuous (Fig. 270).

Figure 271 brings out the irregularity of the lobular reticulin network (Wilder, 375 ×). It must be borne in mind that the presence of giant cells is not pathognomonic of neonatal hepatitis; is may also be seen in atresia of the extrahepatic bile ducts (Fig. 257).

GIANT CELL HEPATITIS WITH PARENCHYMAL COLLAPSE

Male weighing 2,250 gm, unknown gestational age, normal twin birth. Admitted at 2 hours of life. Physical examination not remarkable. Managed with standard care and discharged at 12 days.

Readmitted a few days later with gastroenteritis and metabolic acidosis. Culture of feces was positive for enteropathogenic *E. coli*. Eight days later he was discharged as cured, but returned in 10 days with an acute respiratory process. Clinically and radiographically, a diagnosis of bronchopneumonia was made; the infant was in poor general condition and malnourished. Two weeks later he was discharged, only to the readmitted in another 2 weeks with jaundice of 5 days' duration, again in poor general condition, with choluria and partial acholia, vomiting, and fever.

His condition was extremely serious: metabolic acidosis, pH 7, BE −22 mEq/L. Emergency measures were employed, but the infant died 5 hours later.

Histopathologic Examination. The liver was small at 110 gm against a body weight of 3,750 gm. The surface was smooth. On section, the organ was hard and of a green-yellow color with fine stippling.

Microscopically, there is marked alteration of the cellular pattern. The liver cells are transformed into cellular plasmodia with multiple nuclei. Many cells show necrosis, and there is interspersed round cell infiltration (Figure 272, H & E, 375 ×).

Reticulin stain shows some of the giant cells in the midst of areas of parenchymal collapse where the normal trabecular arrangement is lost. It is as though nests of cells were outlined by areas of collapse.

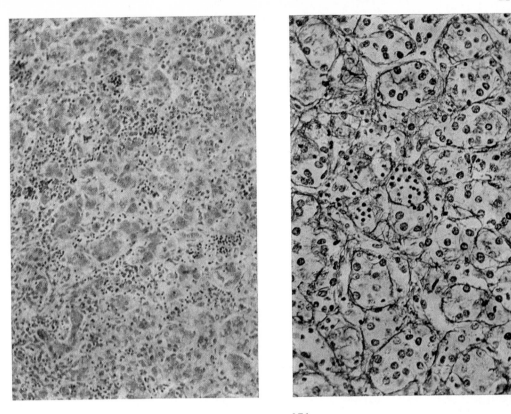

270

271

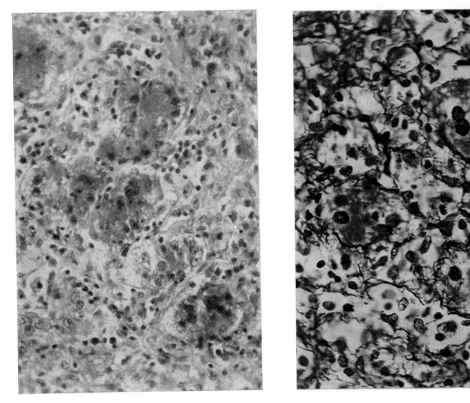

272

273

ACUTE NECROSIS OF THE LIVER

Thirty-day old male, weighing 5,200 gm. Normal delivery. No significant history save for an episode of otititis media 10 days earlier, treated energetically with antibiotics.

Six days prior to admission, fever and restlessness appeared, and again a diagnosis of otitis media was made. Chloramphenicol suppositories were prescribed by the family physician. For 48 hours before admission the infant was deeply jaundiced, and the urine was highly pigmented. On emergency admission, he was in poor general condition with depressed vital signs, obtunded, reacting poorly to stimuli, and vomiting coffee-ground material. The liver was down 1 fingerbreadth. Total bilirubin 8.5 mg/100 ml, direct 6.5 mg/100 ml, microhematocrit 33 per cent, hemoglobin 8.5 gm/100 ml, SGOT 450 u/L, SGPT 650 u/L, total proteins 6.5 gm/100 ml, albumin 4.29 gm/100 ml, gamma globulin 2.04 gm/100 ml. Blood and spinal fluid cultures were negative. EEG showed a well-integrated baseline tracing, with periodic appearance of slow, medium voltage elements at 2–1 c/s. In the following hours his condition worsened; his sensorium deteriorated. In spite of resuscitation, he died as an exchange transfusion was being started.

Histopathologic Examination. The liver weighed 108 gm, and its surface was smooth. The firmness was slightly increased, and the cut surface was yellow with brown stippling, each patch bordered by a gray zone.

Microscopically, the parenchyma appears disorganized and necrotic with persistence of only isolated liver cells and bile ducts (Figure 274 H & E, 187.5 ×).

Greater magnification shows necrotic cells with vacuolated cytoplasm and pale nuclei or none at all. There are also cells with markedly acidophilic cytoplasm and pyknotic nuclei with dense chromatin. The entire area is infiltrated by round cells and some granulocytes (Fig. 275, H & E, 375 ×).

Figure 276 shows obvious irregularity in the distribution of alkaline phosphatase, with increased enzyme activity in the vicinity of the portal areas (375 ×).

Figure 277 reveals the distribution of acid phosphatase, which predominates in the areas of inflammatory infiltration (187.5 ×).

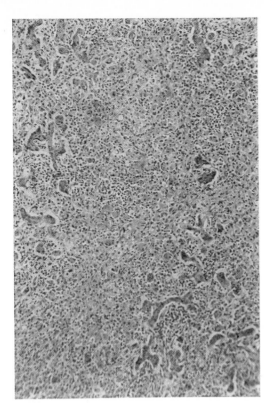

274

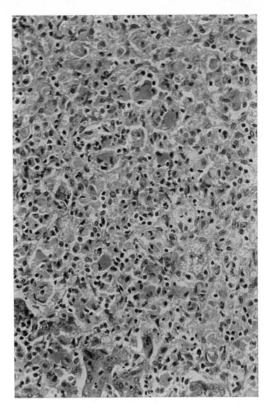

275

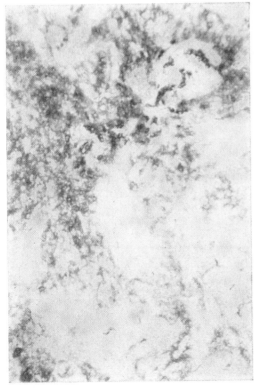

276

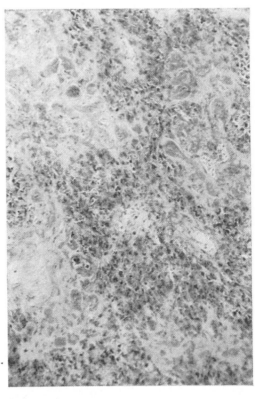

277

278/279
HERPES SIMPLEX SEPSIS

Seven day old male weighing 2.850 gm. Unknown gestational age. Same case as in Figure 215.

Histopathologic Examination. At autopsy the liver was moderately enlarged, weighing 138 gm as against a normal of 105 gm. On the outer surface and on section it showed multiple, diffusely scattered, grayish foci each the size of a pinhead. Microscopically, there were many pale-staining areas, round and well defined, in which liver cells showed advanced necrosis (Fig. 278, H & E, 60 ×).

With greater magnification, many nuclei containing centrally placed, intensely acidophilic inclusion bodies can be seen at the edges of the areas of necrosis. The cytoplasm of these cells is poorly outlined. Above and to the left, a cell is shown that has changed into a globular hyaline mass (Fig. 279, H & E, 1,500 ×).

Similar granulomas were seen in the esophagus (Fig. 215) and the adrenals (Figs. 312 and 313).

The presence of inclusion bodies together with areas of necrosis without inflammatory reaction suggests herpes simplex infection even without identification of the virus.

280
CYTOMEGALIC INCLUSION HEPATITIS

Male weighing 2,800 gm, born at term. Gestational age, 40 weeks. Admitted at 5 hours of life in poor general condition, with jaundice, purpura and hepatosplenomegaly.

A previous sibling was stillborn. During the few weeks preceding delivery the mother suffered from a fever of unknown origin. The amniotic fluid was noted to be brown and to have a fetid odor.

On examination, the infant's sensorium was clear, but there were few spontaneous movements. Myoclonic seizures involving the extremities, a purpuric rash particularly on the trunk, obvious jaundice, and marked hepatosplenomegaly. Laboratory studies ruled out isoimmunization.

Microhematocrit 60 per cent; total bilirubin at 8 hours, 25 mg/100 ml, for which an exchange transfusion was carried out; Hb 10.3 gm/100 ml, 39 per cent erythroblasts; WBC 12,900; platelets 110,000; pH 7.33; pCO_2 38 mm Hg; BE −5.5 mEq/L. Spinal fluid was hemorrhagic, but negative on culture. Urine and blood cultures were negative.

Meconium was cultured on special media for *Listeria,* with negative results. Examination of bone marrow and peripheral blood ruled out congenital leukemia, and two studies for cytomegalic cells in the urine were negative. Serologic testing for syphilis was negative. Examination of the eyegrounds revealed a hemorrhage in the left papilla. X-rays of chest, skull, and skeleton were negative. Dextrose solution with corticoids and antibiotics was administered. After 24 hours there was no change in the patient's course and the myoclonic seizures worsened. At 36 hours of life the infant died.

Histopathologic Examination. Figure 280 shows a small granuloma in the liver. It consists of round monocytoid cells, an occasional granulocyte, and a hepatic cell with a very large nucleus containing a central deeply basophilic inclusion with a clear halo (H & E, 600 ×). The finding of cytomegalic cells in the liver in cases of systemic cytomegalic inclusion disease is not very frequent in our experience, although inflammatory foci may be found.

There were also numerous cytomegalic cells in the lungs, spleen, kidneys, thymus, and brain. The latter showed multiple areas of calcification. There was also an infratentorial hemorrhage and there were visceral petechiae.

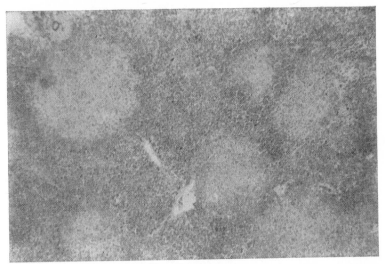

278

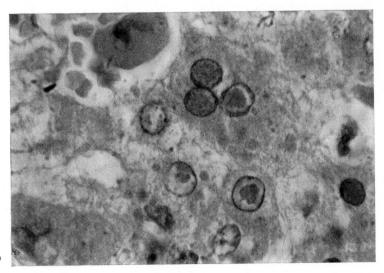

279

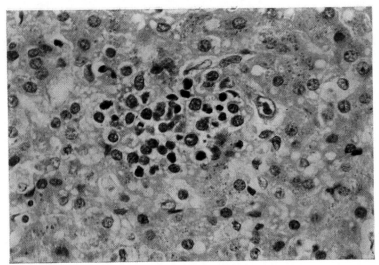

280

281
GRANULOMATOUS CANDIDA HEPATITIS

Male, born at term weighing 3,280 gm. Admitted at 7 days of life because of diarrhea and refusal to feed.

Physical examination: Temperature 39° C, poor general condition, pallor, abdominal distention, and perioral cyanosis. Stools were liquid. There was moderate sclerema of the extremities. The infant appeared dehydrated. Arterial blood pH 7.15, pCO_2 38 mm Hg, BE -14.5 mEq/L, microhematocrit 54 per cent, hemoglobin 17.1 gm/100 ml, total protein 4.0 gm/100 ml.

Treatment for dehydration and acidosis was instituted.

On admission, blood culture on solid medium (Schottmuller plate) showed 261 colonies of enteropathogenic *E. coli*, sensitive to cephalothin, rifampicin, and carbenicillin, per milliliter of cultured blood. Stool cultures were negative for *E. coli*, *Salmonella*, and *Candida*, but showed many colonies of *Staphylococcus*. For 2 days the infant improved with antibiotic treatment and hydration. Then respiratory difficulty set in, and his general condition deteriorated rapidly. Chest x-ray showed micronodular parahilar confluent shadows. Twenty-four hours later he died.

Histopathologic Examination. Figure 281 shows a granuloma in the liver consisting of round cells and granulocytes and containing many hyphae and spores of *Candida*, which stain red with PAS (600 ×).

There were also *Candida* granulomas in the intestine and spleen. The lungs showed scattered hemorrhagic foci.

282/283
LISTERIA HEPATITIS

Male weighing 2,000 gm. Unknown gestational age. Vertex delivery with rupture of membranes 6 hours before.

Admitted at 10 hours of life because of respiratory arrest, generalized cyanosis, hypertonicity, hepatomegaly, poor general condition, and disseminated petechiae. Chest x-ray showed bilateral confluent micronodular shadows. There was conjunctival exudate.

Umbilical vein blood, conjunctival secretions, gastric contents, and spinal fluid were cultured. All were positive for type IV *Listeria*. Death occurred 5 hours after admission.

Histopathologic Examination. At autopsy the liver appeared seeded with well-defined yellow punctate lesions. Microscopically, these lesions are granulomas containing monocytes and abundant cellular necrotic debris. The parenchyma shows stasis and small foci of hematopoiesis (Fig. 282, H & E, 375 ×).

In Figure 283 one of these lesions is illustrated (Levaditi stain); it brings out numerous pleomorphic bacilli within the granulomas (1,500 ×).

There were also *Listeria* granulomas in the meninges, spleen, adrenals, lymph nodes, myocardium, and lungs. Both lungs showed aspiration of meconium and amniotic debris.

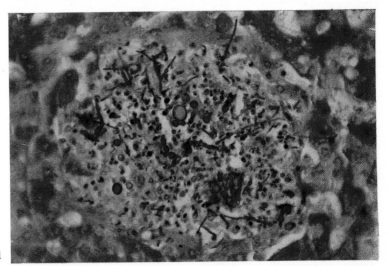

281

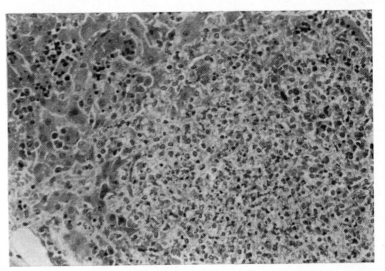

282

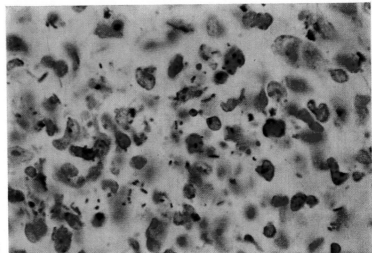

283

284
PSEUDOMONAS SEPSIS

Male weighing 1,080 gm. Gestational age, 32 weeks. Vertex delivery with rupture of membranes 2 hours before. Admitted at 6 hours of life in poor general condition, transported from another city.

On admission there was hypothermia, grayish pallor, and hypotonia. The infant was placed in an incubator.

Studies: pH 7.26, pCO_2 57 mm Hg, BE —4 mEq/L. Chest x-ray showed no significant changes. Blood culture was taken.

The following day the infant's general condition seemed worse. Respiratory difficulty had appeared. A new chest x-ray showed a dense reticulonodular web with confluent areas. pH 6.83 pCO_2 over 100 mm Hg, BE —13.5 mEq/L. Intravenous 1 M bicarbonate solution was started. Death supervened after several bouts of respiratory arrest. The blood culture was positive for *Pseudomonas aeruginosa*.

Histopathologic Examination. At autopsy the liver showed a few yellowish nodules, each well defined and the size of a millet seed. Figure 284 illustrates one of these. The centrolobular vein shows a normal wall on the right, but on the left the wall is necrotic and contains many aggregates of organisms. The nearby liver parenchyma is necrotic; note, however. the absence of any inflammatory reaction in this area (H & E, 375 ×).

Similar necrotic foci were found in the myocardium. The lungs showed granulocytic pneumonia with multiple thrombi in large vessels. Postmortem cultures were positive for *Pseudomonas aeruginosa*.

285
HEMATOGENOUS HEPATIC ABSCESSES IN GENERALIZED SEPSIS

Full-term male weighing 3,350 gm. Rupture of membranes 36 hours before delivery. Apgar score 4 at 1 minute after birth, requiring resuscitation. Admitted at 3 days of life because of deep jaundice, in poor general condition, with respiratory distress. Chest x-ray showed confluent infiltrative shadows, more marked on the right side. Metabolic acidosis. Total bilirubin 22.5 mg/100 ml. Laboratory studies ruled out Rh or ABO isoimmunization.

Blood for culture was taken prior to exchange transfusion, which was done 24 hours later in the face of a persistent elevated bilirubin titer of 23 mg/100 ml. The general condition continued to be grave, with multiple respiratory arrests requiring resuscitation. Death followed in 24 hours. The blood culture was positive for *Klebsiella pneumoniae*.

Histopathologic Examination. Figure 285 shows a section of liver parenchyma with abscesses, some well circumscribed, harboring clusters of organisms. These abscesses are in the immediate vicinity of a longitudinally sectioned vessel, which shows marked inflammatory infiltration of its wall. The remainder of the liver parenchyma shows dilated sinusoids with abundant inflammatory cells in their lumina (H & E, 60 ×).

The infant also had aspirated large amounts of amniotic fluid, and there were many germ-laden necrotic abscesses about the periphery of the lung.

286
FATTY LIVER

Male weighing 2,600 gm. Unknown gestational age. Admitted at 9 days of life for respiratory distress, intercostal retraction, and perioral cyanosis. Examination revealed dehydration; 2 fingerbreadth hepatomegaly; firm, wine red parotid swelling bilaterally; Down's syndrome; and signs of congenital heart disease. Chest x-ray showed the presence of considerable cardiomegaly as well as disseminated and confluent shadows indicating alveolar pulmonary flooding. pH 7.18, pCO_2 47 mm Hg, BE —14 mEq/L. Blood culture was done. There were repeated bouts of respiratory arrest. With oxygen, correction of acidosis, and antibiotic treatment, the child's condition improved temporarily. Two days later, however, there were renewed episodes of apnea, and signs of sepsis returned. He died at 12 days. The blood culture was positive for *E. coli*.

Histopathologic Examination. Figure 286 represents a specimen of liver stained with Sudan III. The trabeculae are well preserved, and the sinusoids are wide. The hepatocytes show, in their cytoplasm, considerable deposition of fat droplets, predominantly in the vicinity of the portal areas (375 ×).

Other autopsy findings: Bilateral suppurative parotitis, diffuse granulocytic pneumonia, and a small, high interventricular septal defect.

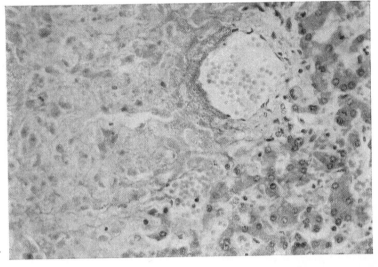

284

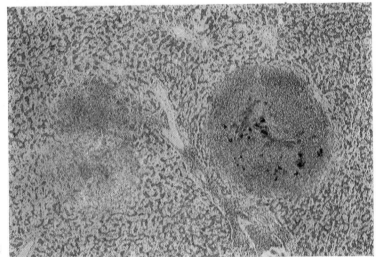

285

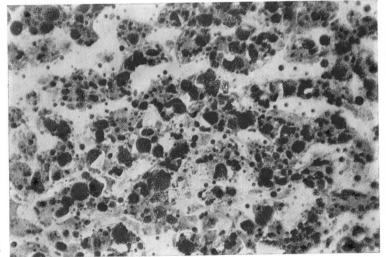

286

LIVER IN CYSTIC FIBROSIS OF THE PANCREAS

Twenty-six day old male weighing 3,150 gm, born at term. Admitted for respiratory difficulty and edema. Physical findings included poor general condition, dehydration, edema of lower extremities, rapid breathing, and fluttering nostrils, but there was no splenic or liver enlargement.

Chest x-ray showed bilateral infiltration, more marked on the right, where it tended toward uniform consolidation. Areas of emphysema were also evident.

Mixed metabolic and respiratory acidosis. Total protein 3.2 gm/100 ml. Urine negative for albumin. Stools moderately diarrheic with a putrid odor. Electrolyte determination in sweat showed increased chloride and sodium; a diagnosis of cystic fibrosis of the pancreas with pulmonary involvement was established. Cultures of pharyngeal exudate and gastric contents were positive for coagulase-positive *Staphylococcus*. A week later respiratory insufficiency developed, followed by disseminated bronchopneumonia and, within 3 days, death.

Histopathologic Examination. The liver weighed 145 gm and was yellowish. Figure 287 shows marked, large droplet fatty metamorphosis of liver cells. On the left there is a portal area with fibrosis and proliferation of dilated bile ducts filled with eosinophilic, partly clumped material that is PAS-positive (375 ×).

The remainder of the autopsy was typical for cystic fibrosis of the pancreas. In addition, there was necrotizing pneumonia, from which cultures yielded *E. coli* and coagulase-positive Staphylococcus.

In children with this disease who survive early infancy, manifestations of portal hypertension may appear because of biliary cirrhosis. The important findings in the biopsy are the presence of bile duct proliferation and especially the presence of mucinous material in dilated ducts. Grossly, the liver may present marked lobulation, similar to that described as "hepar lobatum."

LIVER IN GALACTOSEMIA

Female weighing 2,950 gm. Unknown gestational age. Admitted at 10 days because of diarrhea. Examination showed severe dehydration and prostration, altered sensorium, perioral cyanosis, liquid feces, vomiting, and refusal to feed.

Liquid diet and rehydration were prescribed. Urine positive for albumin and sugar. pH 7.23, pCO_2 39.5 mm Hg, BE −10.5 mEq/L, chloride 140 mEq/L, sodium 179. Treatment for acidosis and hypertonic dehydration. Microhematocrit 68 per cent, total protein 7.2 gm/100 ml, potassium 6.4 mEq/L.

For 2 days the infant improved. Microhematocrit 47 per cent, pH 7.3, pCO_2 46 mm Hg, BE −4 mEq/L, chloride 106 mEq/L, sodium 150 mEq/L, potassium 4.8 mEq/L. Negative stool culture. Negative urine culture.

Onset of respiratory distress. The infant did not tolerate attempts to restore oral feeding, but had vomiting and diarrhea. The liver became palpable. Sugar in the urine was identified as galactose, and there was marked hyperaminoaciduria.

Study of enzymes confirmed the diagnosis of galactosemia. Ten days later the infant died.

Histopathologic Examination. At autopsy the liver weighed 302 gm, showed a smooth surface, a greenish-yellow color, and a soft consistency.

Figure 288 corresponds to an early stage of this disease. The portal area is still normal in size. The surrounding parenchyma shows an architectural change consisting of a tendency to pseudoacinar transformation. There are some bile thrombi in the lumina of these false acini (H & E, 375 ×).

There is considerable fatty change of the parenchyma, as evidenced by Sudan III stain (Fig. 289, 375 ×).

Bronchopneumonia was present in both lungs.

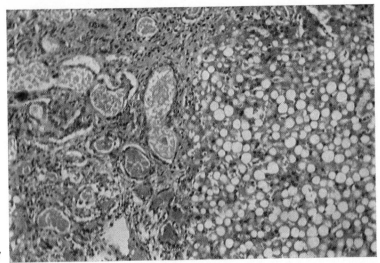

287

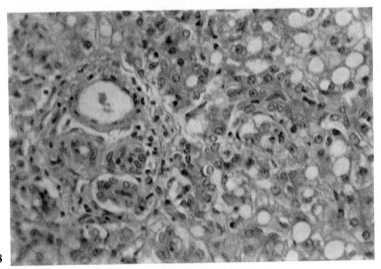

288

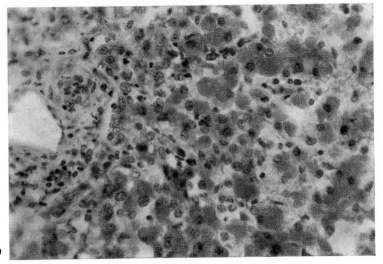

289

290/291
THROMBOSIS OF HEPATIC ARTERY WITH FOCAL LIVER NECROSIS

Male weighing 2,760 gm, born at term by cesarean section. Admitted at 8 hours because of respiratory difficulty. There were hypothermia, cyanosis, superficial and irregular breathing, and a very weak cry. Examination revealed marked loss of tone, absence of spontaneous movements, tachypnea, intercostal retraction, and the beginning of pseudo-pectus excavatum. Chest x-ray showed reticulogranular shadows and air bronchogram. Blood was obtained by catheterization of the umbilical artery and vein for studies: arterial pH 7.21, pCO_2 60 mm Hg, BE -8 mEq/L, pO_2 while in 45 per cent oxygen 18 mm Hg, hemoglobin saturation 58 per cent. Infusion of 10 per cent glucose and 1 M bicarbonate was given.

Six hours later, subcostal inspiratory tug persisted. pH 7.24, pCO_2 64 mm Hg, BE -4 mEq/L, pO_2 in 100 per cent oxygen 66 mm Hg. Frequent apneic crises requiring resuscitation continued. On the sixth day generalized sclerema appeared and was followed by vomiting of fresh blood, which necessitated aspiration of the airway. Death occurred that day.

The diagnosis was hyaline membrane disease with pulmonary hemorrhage and sclerema. Cultures of feces, gastric contents, and blood were negative.

Histopathologic Examination. Figure 290 shows a hilar intrahepatic branch of the hepatic artery at the point where the tip of a catheter was lodged. Note the presence of a parietal fibrinoleukocytic thrombus that is continuous with the wall (H & E, 187.5 ×). The liver showed a number of areas of necrosis.

Figure 291 shows a hemorrhagic area of necrosis adjacent to an area of normal parenchyma (H & E, 375 ×).

Other findings included the presence of a residual picture of hyaline membranes in the process of resorption and associated inflammatory lesions.

292/293
LIVER IN TRIPLOIDY

Male weighing 2,430 gm. Gestational age, 40 weeks; cesarean delivery. Case corresponds also to Figures 121 and 188 to 191.

Histopathologic Examination. The trabecular architecture of the liver is normal, but the size of the nuclei shown in Figure 292 and particularly the dense and granular appearance of the nuclear chromatin are conspicuously different from that of the normal liver in Figure 293 (H & E, 600 ×).

The average diameter of the nuclei in this case of triploidy was 8.937 ± 0.075 microns, statistically significantly different from those in a control group of newborns of the same weight.

Other autopsy findings included hydrocephalus, agenesis of the corpus callosum, adrenal hypoplasia, fibrosis of the myocardium (Fig. 121), congenital glomerulosclerosis with unilateral renal dysplasia (Figs. 188 to 191), and hyperplasia of Leydig cells.

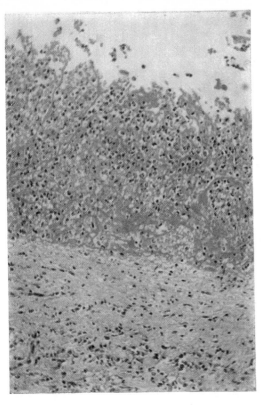

290

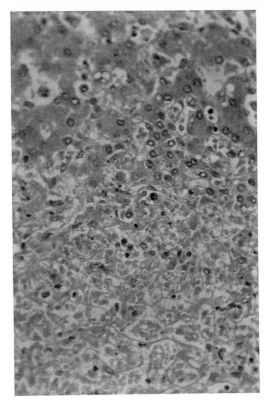

291

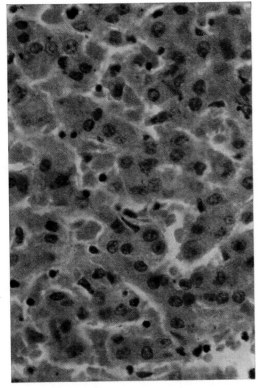

292

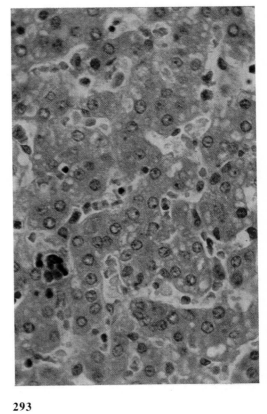

293

294
CAVERNOUS HEMANGIOMA OF THE LIVER

Male weighing 2,700 gm. Gestational age, 38 weeks. Admitted at 36 hours of life with respiratory distress.

At birth there had been signs of anoxia requiring energetic resuscitation. On admission, cyanosis, rapid respiration, irregular breathing, generalized loss of tone, and mixed metabolic and respiratory acidosis were observed. Chest x-ray showed a pattern suggestive of possible aspiration. Death occurred in a crisis of apnea 4 hours after admission. The liver was palpable 2 fingerbreadths below the costal margin.

Histopathologic Examination. The liver weighed 242 gm and contained a mass that occupied practically the entire right lobe. It was made up of a spongelike network of blood vessels. Figure 294 shows the histologic appearance of the mass, which was made up of large vascular channels separated from one another by delicate connective tissue strands lined by endothelium (H & E, 187.5 ×).

The ultimate cause of death was bronchopneumonia involving all lobes.

295
MESENCHYMAL HAMARTOMA OF THE LIVER

Male weighing 3,500 gm, born at term. Admitted at 28 days of age because of rapid increase of abdominal girth without other symptoms. A mass of moderately firm consistency occupied all of the right upper quadrant. Routine laboratory studies were normal.

X-ray examination showed an area of opacification in the right side of the abdomen displacing intestinal loops downward and toward the left. Cholecystogram revealed displacement of the gallbladder toward the left. In a liver scan carried out with colloidal gold (Au 198) the outline of the liver appeared normal, but there was an abnormal crescent-shaped image with its concavity directed downward, representing a well-defined cold area. The characteristics of the scan did not rule out extrinsic pressure.

At surgery a cystic intrahepatic mass was found, and a partial right hemihepatectomy was performed. The bile ducts and the pancreas were normal. The postoperative course was uneventful, and 20 days later the infant was discharged. Findings at repeated follow-up examinations for the succeeding 2 years were normal.

Histopathologic Examination. The specimen consisted of a grayish-white tumor mass with reddish patches and cystic spaces. Microscopically, it was made up of areas of relatively acellular connective tissue bearing remnants of bile ducts and spaces occupied by fluid.

Figure 295 shows a portion of the wall of one of the cysts, devoid of its epithelial lining, with a fibrinous inner layer. The supporting collagenous connective tissue bears the hemorrhagic area seen in the upper part of the illustration. No atypia was apparent (H & E, 375 ×).

296/297
CONGENITAL NEUROBLASTOMA WITH MASSIVE HEPATIC INVOLVEMENT

Male weighing 3,250 gm, born at term by cesarean section. Admitted 2 hours after birth. (This is the same case as is shown in Figure 225.)

On admission the infant was in poor general condition with pallor, absence of spontaneous movements, and loss of tone. Marked enlargement of the abdomen was obvious and attributable to a giant, palpable tumor mass with a well-defined edge. It extended to within 1 cm of the iliac crest and gave the impression of being part of the liver. No renal enlargement or splenomegaly could be perceived. Microhematocrit 38 per cent, hemoglobin 11.7 gm/100 ml, leukocytes 20,500 cu mm, platelets 15,000/cu mm, pH 7.10, pCO_2 57 mm Hg, BE −13.5 mEq/L, total bilirubin 3.5 mg/100 ml. Acidosis was corrected with dextrose-bicarbonate infusion.

X-ray examination showed obvious lack of pulmonary expansion. Lateral films suggested extrinsic compression. The pyelogram was normal, but showed a delay in excretion on the right side. The umbilical arteriogram showed rapid filling of the pulmonary arteries and the presence of enlarged suprahepatic veins. There were no calcifications in the hepatic region. Death followed a crisis of hypertonicity and disseminated cutaneous petechiae.

Histopathologic Examination. The liver was much enlarged, weighing 640 gm. Its firmness was increased and the tissue was grayish-red without any obvious nodules.

Microscopically, however, there was massive invasion of the organ by neuroblasts with loss or atrophy of the liver cell laminae, which could be identified only in some small areas (Fig. 296, H & E, 375 ×).

Autopsy revealed invasion of the pancreas. The primary tumor arose in the right adrenal. Figure 297 shows the characteristic appearance of neuroblastoma metastatic to the liver in a 25 day old child (H & E 187.5 ×).

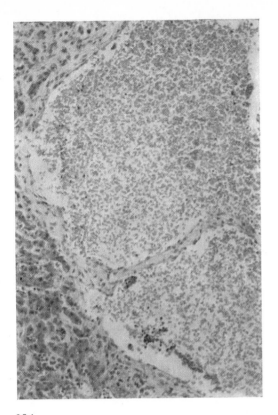

294

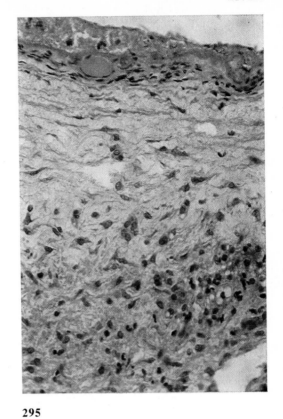

295

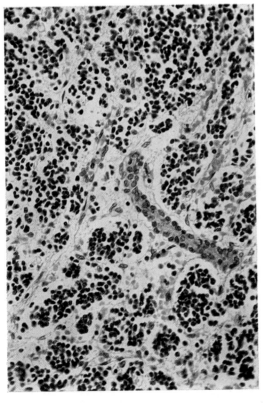

296

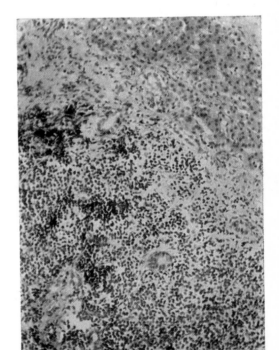

297

Adrenals

298
ECTOPIC ADRENAL TISSUE IN THE OVARY

Female, 3 hours old, weighing 1,500 gm. Gestational age, 26 weeks. Breech presentation, twin birth. Apgar score 2 at 1 minute. Resuscitation required.

On admission there were signs of immaturity and generalized hypotonia. Facial edema. Generalized cyanosis. Metabolic acidosis. Death occurred 4 hours after admission.

Histopathologic Examination. The upper part of Figure 298 shows the ovary (H & E, 60×). On the right there is a nest of aberrant adrenal tissue identical to that shown in Figure 299 (H & E, 60×).

Autopsy showed generalized petechial hemorrhages as well as pulmonary congestion and atelectasis.

299
ECTOPIC ADRENAL TISSUE IN THE TESTICLE

Male weighing 800 gm. Gestational age, 26 weeks. Admitted 8 hours after birth. Examination showed generalized hypotonia, signs of immaturity, and generalized cyanosis. There was mixed metabolic and respiratory acidosis. An episode of respiratory arrest occurred at 2 hours; others followed and the infant died during one of them.

Histopathologic Examination. In the lower part of Figure 299 testicular tissue can be seen, and within the epididymis is a rounded nest of adrenal tissue. The darkly stained external portion corresponds to adult cortex, while the central portion represents fetal cortex (H & E, 60×).

Autopsy showed obvious evidences of immaturity in all organs and early formation of pulmonary hyaline membranes.

300
ADRENORENAL FUSION

Twenty-six day old female admitted for acute respiratory insufficiency. Weight: 2,250 gm. Gestational age unknown. On admission, Down's syndrome with atrioventricularis communis was diagnosed. The infant's general condition was poor. Chest x-ray showed infiltration in the right suprahilar region. There were areas

of emphysema and cardiac enlargement. In spite of treatment with digitalis and antibiotics, death occurred 24 hours later. pH 7.29, pCO_2 54 mm Hg, BE −7 mEq/L.

Histopathologic Examination. In the upper part of Figure 300 is shown adrenal tissue (corresponding to the left adrenal) with fibrosis and dilated vessels in close proximity to the renal parenchyma with no intervening capsule. There are no significant changes in either of the two types of parenchyma (Masson, 60 ×).

In this case there was also adrenohepatic fusion on the right.

Autopsy demonstrated the presence of the aforementioned congenital cardiac anomaly and a moderate degree of bronchopneumonia.

301
ADRENOHEPATIC FUSION

Male weighing 2,160 gm. Gestational age, 36 weeks. Product of a sixth twin birth. Admitted 3 days after delivery with diarrhea and marked abdominal distention. Signs of respiratory insufficiency. Physical examination disclosed the presence of Down's syndrome, bronchopneumonia, and a congenital cardiac anomaly. General condition was poor. Cultures of urine and gastric contents yielded *Klebsiella*. Chest x-ray showed the presence of cardiac enlargement and bilateral bronchopneumonia. In 2 days abdominal distention increased, and diarrhea alternated with periods of constipation. Barium enema showed the presence of megacolon.

There was a pansystolic murmur. Cardiologic examination reinforced the diagnostic impression of interventricular septal defect. Death occurred 5 days after admission.

Histopathologic Examination. Figure 301 shows, on the left, liver parenchyma in direct continuity with the fetal zone of the adrenal cortex without any intervening capsule. The line of fusion is irregular, but there is no reaction nor is there any architectural change in the parenchymal cells of either organ (H & E, 60×).

This developmental anomaly is relatively rare. We have observed it only three times in 2,500 autopsies of children between the ages of 0 and 7 years. In the 3 cases it was found in children with Down's syndrome.

Autopsy showed the presence of an interventricular septal defect, aganglionic megacolon, ulcerative enterocolitis, and bilateral bronchopneumonia.

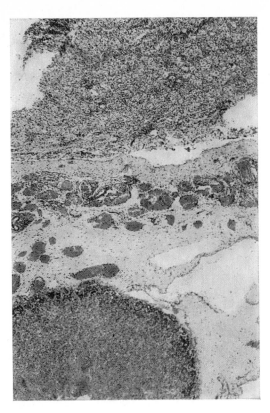

298

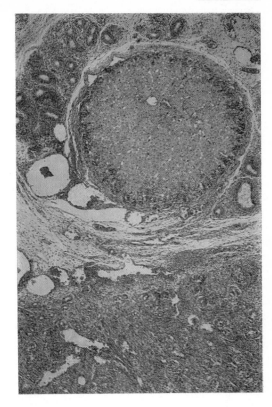

299

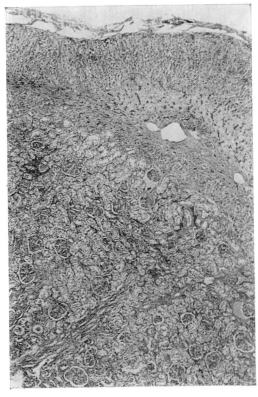

300

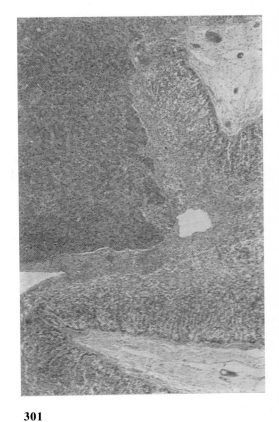

301

302
PSEUDOCYSTIC TRANSFORMATION OF THE ADRENAL

Male weighing 700 gm. Gestational age, 26 weeks. Born by vertex presentation. Apgar score 2 at birth. Resuscitation required.

Admitted 1 hour after birth. General immaturity was apparent on physical examination, with cyanosis, areflexia, and signs of respiratory insufficiency.

Two hours later respiratory arrest occurred, and the infant died in spite of attempts at resuscitation.

Histopathologic Examination. Figure 302 shows adrenal cortex with numerous empty cystic spaces along the periphery. There is marked congestion of the fetal cortex (H & E, 187.5 ×).

A similar picture can be observed in pseudotubular transformation in children dying of septicemia with secondary cortical atrophy.

Autopsy showed generalized immaturity and pulmonary anectasia.

303
ADRENAL HYPOPLASIA

Female weighing 3,100 gm, born at term. Admitted 2 hours after birth because of anencephaly. Signs of respiratory insufficiency were present, and in the 10 hours following admission there were repeated bouts of respiratory arrest during one of which the infant died.

Histopathologic Examination. Both adrenals were small: combined weight 1 gm. They were normally located. Microscopic examination of the adrenal demonstrates resemblance to mature adrenal with the absence of any fetal zone. Microscopic architecture is otherwise normal and there are no megalocytes (H & E, 60 ×).

Autopsy showed aplasia of the bones of the cranial vault. There was a 5 cm flat mass of tissue on the base of the skull, covered by skin and consisting of connective tissue with vessels and cavities containing clear fluid. There was extensive pulmonary atelectasis.

304
CONGENITAL ADRENAL HYPERPLASIA

Sixteen day old male. At birth he weighed 4,000 gm. Gestational age, 38 weeks. Breast fed. Admitted because of repeated vomiting and poor general condition.

Physical examination showed signs of moderate dehydration, poor general condition, acidosis, and an earthy pallor. The size of the penis was slightly increased. X-ray of the chest showed moderate perihilar infiltrates. pH 7.17, pCO_2 41 mm Hg, BE −16.5 mEq/L. Acidosis was corrected with the administration of intravenous bicarbonate. Sodium 125 mEq/L, potassium 4.5 mEq/L, chlorides 98 mEq/L.

After his respiratory distress diminished he vomited continuously. Examinations of the digestive system were, however, normal. Four days after admission there was a sudden episode of collapse with dehydration, severe loss of tone, and metabolic acidosis requiring urgent therapeutic measures. Signs of respiratory insufficiency continued, and the chest x-ray showed bilateral patchy consolidation. Determination of 17-ketosteroids and pregnanetriol in the urine collected for 24 hours allowed for confirmation of the diagnosis of congenital adrenal hyperplasia. Appropriate treatment was instituted. The respiratory systems became worse, however, and the patient died 3 days later.

Histopathologic Examination. Autopsy showed bilateral adrenal enlargement. Both glands together weighed 14 gm. The surface of each had an encephaloid appearance with extracortical nodules as shown in Figure 304 (H & E, 15 ×). Histologic architecture was regular and represented mature (nonfetal) cortex.

Autopsy showed the presence of bilateral interstitial pneumonia with hyaline membranes.

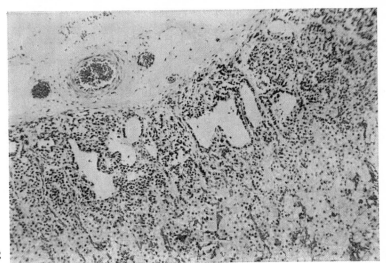

302

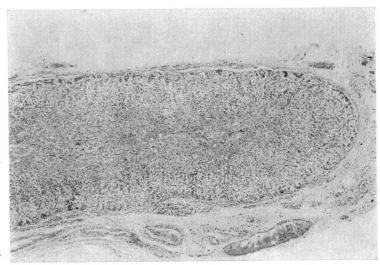

303

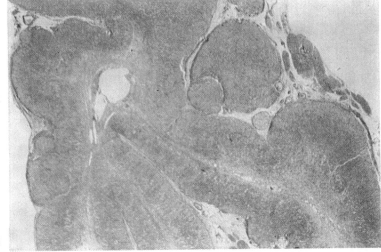

304

305/306/307
CONGENITAL LIPOID HYPERPLASIA OF FETAL ZONE

Female weighing 1,750 gm. Gestational age, 30 weeks. Apgar score 4. Admitted 10 minutes after delivery. Marked pallor. Very poor general condition. Respiratory arrest occurred. Microhematocrit 15 per cent. Blood group O, Rh positive; mother O, Rh positive. A transfusion of 40 ml of blood was carried out immediately; 1 M bicarbonate and 10 per cent dextrose were administered. Respiratory arrest continued, and the patient died 4 hours after admission. The clinical diagnosis was acute anemia due to probable fetoplacental transfusion and respiratory insufficiency.

Histopathologic Examination. At autopsy there was marked pallor of all viscera. The genitalia were normal female. On microscopic examination, there was extensive pulmonary atelectasis.

Adrenals were enlarged, with a combined weight of 10.5 gm (normal for the body weight, 4.3 gm). The relationship between mature cortex and fetal cortex was 1:12 instead of 1:4, which is normal.

On section, there was diffuse and marked yellow discoloration. Figure 305 shows the appearance of the fetal zone of the adrenal with a Wilder reticulin stain. There is no collapse of the reticulum network, and the cells are large and vesicular (375 ×).

With Sudan III stain, there is an obvious and abundant deposition of neutral fats in the cytoplasm of these cells (Fig. 306, 375 ×).

Under polarized light, a marked accumulation of birefringent lipids is demonstrated (Fig. 207, 375 ×).

In a series of 1,432 infant autopsies we observed this type of lipid deposition in the fetal zone of the adrenal in 2 cases (0.14 per cent). One of them is the case just described. The second was a 3,400 gm newborn with erythroblastosis due to Rh incompatibility Although the significance of this lesion is not clear, it is possible that it may be related to severe anemia of the newborn. The deposition of lipid in the adrenals of children dying with hemolytic anemia has been described, and there seems to be some correlation between the amount of lipid deposition and the degree of anemia. On the other hand, there is no correlation with the weight of the adrenals.

This picture of excessive lipid deposition within the fetal zone of the adrenal must not be confused with congenital hyperplasia of the adrenal.

182

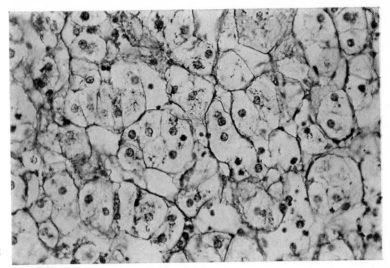

305

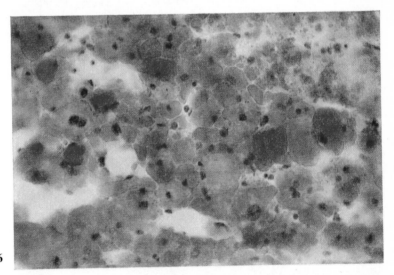

306

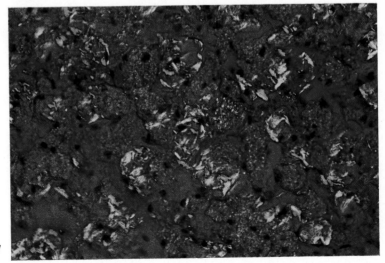

307

308
ADRENAL CALCIFICATION

A 15 day old female weighing 3,600 gm. Admitted because of generalized desquamative dermatopathy and acute respiratory distress.

Additional studies showed the presence of bronchopneumonia, hypoproteinemia, and hypogammaglobulinemia. Immunoelectrophoresis showed normal values for IgA and IgG and the absence of IgM. Cultures of nasal secretions and pharyngeal secretions were positive for *Pseudomonas aeruginosa* and *Proteus mirabilis*. Pulmonary changes became progressively worse, and the infant's general condition deteriorated; death followed on the fourth day after admission.

Histopathologic Examination. The architecture of the adrenal cortex is normal. In the corticomedullary junction is observed a broad zone of calcification with coarse deposits of calcium, irregularly arranged and, deeper, a band of loose connective tissue (H & E, 187.5 ×). We interpret this as dystrophic calcification based on a probable previous hemorrhage within the adrenals.

Autopsy showed necrotizing bronchopneumonia. There was exfoliative dermatitis accompanied by fatty change in the liver and involution of the thymus. There were no anomalous deposits of cholesterol.

309
ADRENAL NECROSIS

Male weighing 3,350 gm, born at term by vertex presentation. Apgar score 10 at birth. Admitted 2 days later because of deep jaundice and respiratory difficulty.

On admission, the infant's general condition was poor with irregular respirations and intercostal retraction. Jaundice was obvious. Hematocrit 52 per cent, total bilirubin 16.5 mg/100 ml, direct Coomb's test negative. X-ray of the chest showed areas of consolidation in the right lung field. In the succeeding hours the patient's general condition deteriorated and the clinical picture of generalized sepsis appeared. Four hours later the child died.

Blood culture taken at the time of admission was negative.

Histopathologic Examination. Figure 309 shows a significant area of necrosis of adrenal tissue with partial fibrinoid change. At its junction with preserved tissue there is a capillary containing a hyaline thrombus, the wine-red

color of which contrasts with the pink of the necrotic portion. Note the absence of inflammatory cells in the area (H & E, 187.5 ×).

Autopsy also showed aspiration of amniotic debris with phagocytic reaction of the alveolar lining cells as well as septal pulmonary hemorrhages, interstitial hemorrhage in the testicle and myocardium, and hyaline thrombi in the vessels of the myocardium, bladder, and spleen.

310/311
ADRENAL CYTOMEGALY

Female weighing 1,490 gm. Gestational age, 28 weeks. Admitted 3 hours after birth because of respiratory difficulty, whining, generalized cyanosis, edema of the scalp, marked generalized hypotonia, and apneic episodes. Spinal tap yielded hemorrhagic fluid. Repeated crises of respiratory arrest and cyanosis eventuated in death 19 hours after admission.

Histopathologic Examination. Figure 310 shows a portion of the fetal zone of the adrenal, including large cells with granular, sharply outlined cytoplasm with some lighter areas. The nuclei are enlarged and chromatin is abundant (H & E, 600 ×).

Stained with Sudan III, these cells show considerable deposition of lipids (Fig. 311, 600 ×).

This lesion, the significance of which is unknown, should not be confused with the cellular changes seen in cytomegalovirus infection (Fig. 315). This type of megalocytosis associated with hypoplasia of the adrenal has been described in omphalocele-macroglossia-visceromegaly-hypoglycemia, or Beckwith's, syndrome.

Autopsy also showed bilateral interventricular hemorrhage as the cause of death, with hemorrhages into the substance of the brain and the meninges.

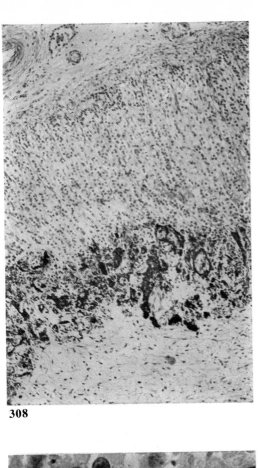

308

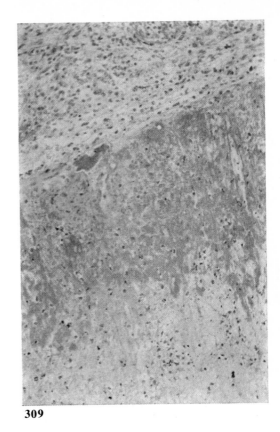

309

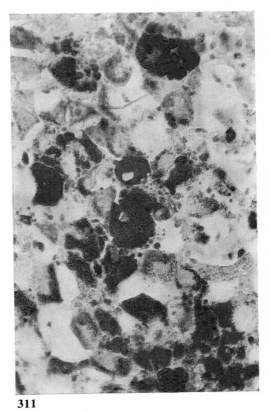

310

311

312/313
ADRENAL HERPES SIMPLEX INFECTION

Male weighing 2,850 gm. Unknown gestational age. This is the same case as is shown in Figures 215, 278, and 279.

Histopathologic Examination. Figure 312 shows a part of the adrenal cortex. The capsule appears in the upper right corner. Under the capsule there is a zone made up of unusually clear cells and rounded foci of necrosis with some cellular debris in the center. Note the absence of any inflammatory component within this area or in adjacent normal tissue (H & E, 375 ×).

In the vicinity of this area, some of the intact adrenal cells show intranuclear inclusions, which are large and eosinophilic, each surrounded by a clear halo that separates it from the thickened nuclear membrane (Fig. 313, H & E, 1,500 ×).

Similar lesions were seen in the liver (Figs. 278 and 279) and in the esophagus (Fig. 215).

314
ADRENAL IN LISTERIOSIS

Male weighing 2,730 gm. Gestational age, 32 weeks. Admitted 44 hours after delivery with respiratory insufficiency, generalized sepsis, earthy pallor, generalized hypertonicity, hepatosplenomegaly, rhinitis, and generalized petechiae. X-ray of the chest showed confluent micronodular densities in the lungs. Culture of blood obtained by umbilical vein catheterization was positive for *Listeria*, as was that of the meconium.

In spite of intensive treatment the infant died 7 hours after admission.

Histopathologic Examination. At autopsy the adrenal presented a number of whitish nodules, clearly outlined and in sharp contrast to the reddish color of the rest of the parenchyma.

Figure 314 shows the microscopic appearance of one of these areas. A large granuloma in the fetal zone of the cortex has necrotic edges and an occasional focal hemorrhage. The cells in the center of the lesion are mostly monocytes (H & E, 60 ×).

Gram stain showed pleomorphic gram-positive organisms within these lesions.

At autopsy, *Listeria* granulomas were also found in the lungs, adrenals, and kidneys.

315
CYTOMEGALIC INCLUSION DISEASE INVOLVING THE ADRENAL

Female weighing 1,150 gm. Gestational age, 29 weeks. The same case is illustrated in Figures 213 and 229. Detailed clinical history accompanies the latter.

Histopathologic Examination. In the outer layer of the adrenal cortex there are many cytomegalic cells with typical nuclear basophilic inclusions, each surrounded by a clear halo. There is no associated inflammatory infiltration (H & E, 375 ×). Compare this picture with Figure 310.

Similar cytomegalic inclusions were found in the lungs, kidneys, thyroid, intestine, spleen, liver, ovaries, myocardium, esophagus (Fig. 213), and pancreas (Fig. 229).

Other lesions included diffuse interstitial pneumonia, generalized icteric pigmentation, and cholestasis in the liver.

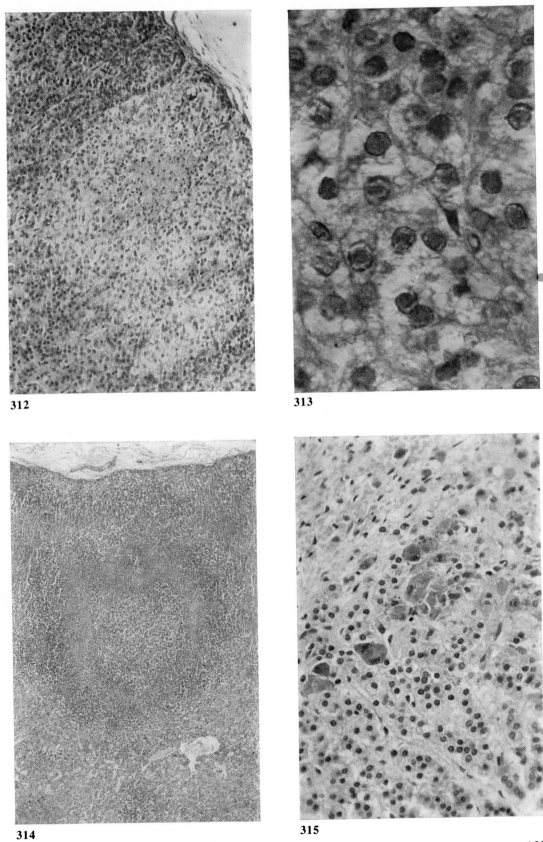

312

313

314

315

316
CANDIDIASIS INVOLVING THE ADRENAL

Female weighing 2,360 gm. Gestational age, 37 weeks. Admitted 3 days after birth because of abundant sialorrhea and cyanosis at the start of feedings. On admission, the infant's general condition was poor and x-rays showed esophageal atresia with tracheoesophageal fistula. X-ray of the lung showed paratracheal infiltration on the right, probably caused by aspiration. Treatment to improve the infant's general condition was instituted, and surgery was carried out 48 hours later. The postoperative course was stormy, with severe respiratory insufficiency. Generalized sepsis appeared. Blood culture was negative; however, cultures of gastric contents and urine were positive for *Klebsiella pneumoniae*. Death occurred at 10 days.

Histopathologic Examination. In the midzone of the adrenal cortex there is a granuloma. PAS stain shows hyphae and spores of *Candida* within it (375 ×).

Similar lesions were found in the liver, spleen, myocardium, lungs, kidney, and brain.

317
CONGENITAL TOXOPLASMOSIS WITH ADRENAL INVOLVEMENT

Female weighing 2,480 gm. Gestational age, 32 weeks. The same case is illustrated in Figures 116, 156 and 157, and 356 and 357.

Histopathologic Examination. The adrenals did not reveal any gross changes. Observed under the microscope, as shown in Figure 317, was a distinct lesion made up of an accumulation of basophilic bodies, sharply circumscribed, in the midst of an area of necrobiosis. These bodies represent *Toxoplasma* organisms. There is no inflammatory infiltration around the accumulation (H & E, 1500 ×).

Granulomatous lesions were also found in the choroid of the eye and the retina (Figs. 356 and 357), myocardium (Fig. 116), and brain (Figs. 156 and 157).

318
HEMORRHAGIC INFARCTION OF THE ADRENAL

Male weighing 3,000 gm, born at term with no significant history until 24 days of life. Twelve hours before admission a high fever was detected. There were continual whining and refusal to feed. Six hours later, pallor was noted, and the infant's condition deteriorated. Admitted as an emergency.

On admission, poor general condition was observed, with perioral cyanosis and acrocyanosis; purpuric spots were scattered throughout. There was severe peripheral vascular collapse with marked hypotension and tachycardia. The abdomen was distended, and there was hepatomegaly. Hematocrit 40 per cent, leukocytes 1,800/cu mm with 90 per cent lymphocytes, platelets 12,000 cu mm, pH 6.99, pCO_2 more than 100 mm Hg. Blood for culture was drawn. In spite of emergency measures the infant continued to do poorly. Laboratory studies showed: hematocrit 40 per cent, total protein 5.2 gm/100 ml, pH 7.09, pCO_2 46 mm Hg, BE −16.5 mEq/L, sodium 148 mEq/L, potassium 5.3 mEq/L, chloride 104 mEq/L. His condition deteriorated, and he died 9 hours later.

Blood culture grew out *Klebsiella*.

Histopathologic Examination. Necropsy showed adrenals of normal size with bilateral marked hemorrhagic infiltration.

Figure 318 shows almost total disappearance of the normal structure of the gland with persistence of some cell cords in the subcapsular zone and complete hemorrhagic disintegration of the remainder (H & E, 375 ×).

There were also petechiae in the myocardium and skin as well as hyaline thrombi in the capillaries of the lung.

319
NEUROBLASTOMA IN SITU

Male born at term weighing 3,000 gm. Normal delivery. From the fourth day of life there were abnormal stools. At 8 days the infant was admitted because of continued liquid bowel movements. Two days before admission progressive respiratory difficulty began. On admission, his general condition was poor, with rapid breathing and dehydration. There was no hepato- or splenomegaly. pH 7.07, pCO_2 26 mm Hg, BE −22 mEq/L, chlorides 138 mEq/L, sodium 151 mEq/L, potassium 5 mEq/L. Chest x-ray showed a small heart and elevation of the right hemidiaphragm. Death occurred 18 hours after admission. Cultures of blood, stool, and gastric contents yielded *E. coli*.

Histopathologic Examination. Figure 319 shows the medullary region of the adrenal to be occupied by densely cellular tissue made up of neuroblasts. There is no apparent invasion of the cortex. In the midst of the mass are a few pseudorosettes (H & E, 60 ×).

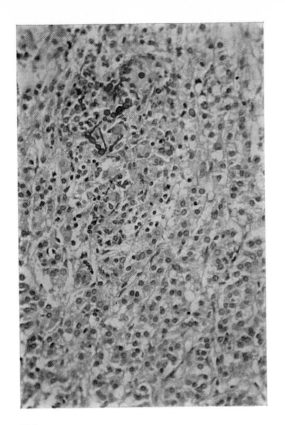

316

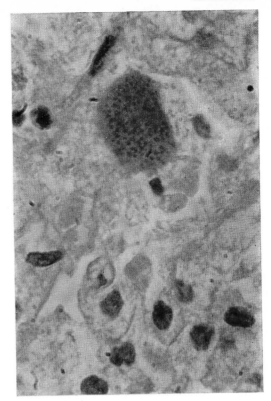

317

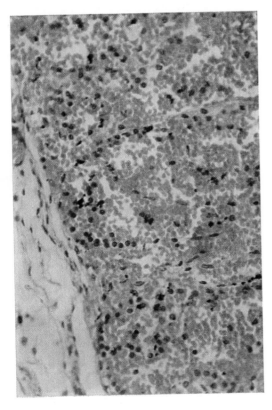

318

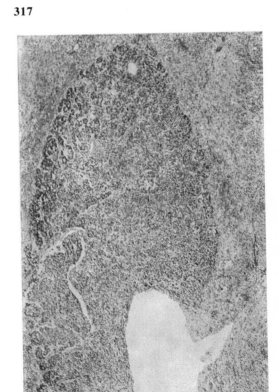

319

Thyroid

320
NUCLEAR AGGREGATES IN THE THYROID OF A NEWBORN

Female weighing 3,150 gm. Gestational age, 41 weeks. Admitted 2 hours after delivery. The amniotic fluid was brownish-green, and there were other clinical signs suggestive of fetal distress. On admission the infant appeared moribund, with considerable loss of tone, gasping, and generalized cyanosis. In spite of intensive treatment with assisted respiration and intubation, she died almost immediately.

Histopathologic Examination. The thyroid appears solid, with clear cells as the principal component. Follicular differentiation is scanty, and there is no colloid (H & E, 375 ×).

Note the presence of numerous nuclear conglomerates forming dense clusters. Emery interprets this pattern as an expression of thyroid discharge. (Translators' note: It may, however, and probably does, represent autolysis.)

At autopsy there were extensive areas of atelectasis in the lung and cystic lymphangiectasias.

321
LINGUAL THYROID. ATHYROIDISM

Twenty-five day old female weighing 4,300 gm, born by cesarean section, with a normal immediate neonatal period. Persistent jaundice was noticeable from birth; the skin, very dry. Abundant hair with low hairline. The facial features typical of hypothyroidism, the presence of an umbilical hernia, and constipation permitted the suspicion of thyroid deficiency, which subsequent studies confirmed. Scan showed the complete absence of thyroid tissue at the expected site.

At 25 days of life a respiratory syndrome developed with progressive insufficiency, metabolic, and respiratory acidosis. The infant died at 28 days.

Histopathologic Examination. At autopsy no thyroid gland could be found in the normal location.

Figure 321 shows a section of the base of the tongue with groups of seromucous glands (on the right side of the illustration). Deeper within the musculature there is a large cyst accompanied by a group of thyroid acini containing scanty colloid (H & E, 60 ×).

Death was due to interstitial pneumonia with some giant cell granulomas. There were also many foci of nephrocalcinosis and cysts of the ovaries.

322
GOITER OF CONGENITAL HYPERTHYROIDISM

Male weighing 2,750 gm, 35 weeks' gestational age, fourth pregnancy. Born by caeserean section. Apgar score 2 at birth. The three preceding siblings had died at birth of unknown causes. This infant was admitted at 3 hours of life in severe respiratory distress. Chest x-rays supported the clinical diagnosis of hyaline membrane disease.

Studies carried out on blood from the umbilical artery revealed very low values for pCO_2 (while the infant was breathing 100 per cent oxygen) and respiratory acidosis. In the midline of the neck, at the level of the epiglottis, there was a small trilobed mass not adherent to the skin or deep tissues. It was considered to be a hypertrophic thyroid. The mother had been operated upon for goiter shortly before this pregnancy.

The infant died 24 hours after admission in respiratory insufficiency.

Histopathologic Examination. The thyroid was clearly enlarged, weighing 11 gm. The cell structure of the gland was reminiscent of the pattern of Graves' disease in the adult. The follicles are large, with irregular configuration, and lined by tall epithelial cells, showing pseudopapillary projections into lumina containing no stainable colloid (H & E, 375 ×).

The lungs showed the histologic characteristics of hyaline membrane disease.

323
"CYSTIC" COLLOID GOITER

Male weighing 2,450 gm. Gestational age, 36 weeks. Admitted at 24 hours of life with respiratory difficulty and generalized cyanosis. Malformations of trisomy 13 corroborated by karyotyping. Radiographic examination showed cardiomegaly with scanty pulmonary vascularization. The respiratory picture worsened progressively, and death occurred 24 hours after admission.

Histopathologic Examination. The thyroid weighed 9 gm. Figure 323 shows thyroid follicles of various sizes, some of them markedly dilated and filled with acidophilic colloid. The follicles are lined by flattened epithelial cells (H & E, 187.5 ×).

Autopsy confirmed that this was a case of trisomy 13 with multiple malformations including a full-blown tetralogy of Fallot. The lungs showed the typical picture of congestive atelectasis and hyaline membrane disease.

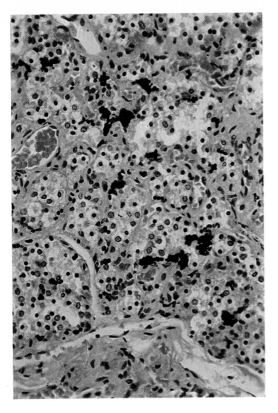

320

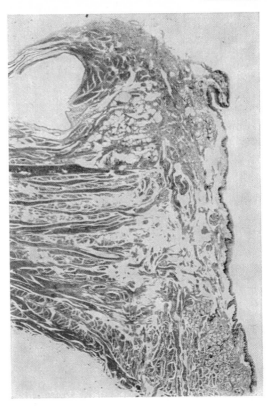

321

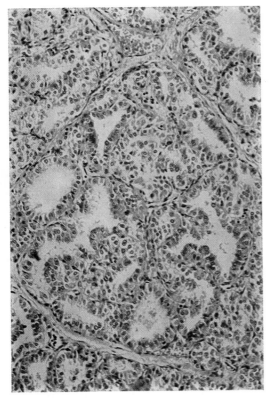

322

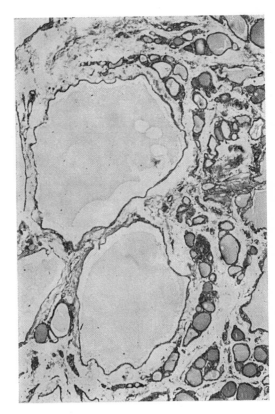

323

Genitalia

324
IMMATURE OVARY

Female weighing 790 gm, 29 weeks' gestational age. Admitted 2 hours after birth showing overt signs of immaturity, respiratory difficulty with cyanosis and rapid breathing, poor general condition. No cardiac murmurs. Coarse facial features and moderate macroglossia. Chest x-ray showed uniform cardiac enlargement but no significant pulmonary changes. Marked loss of muscle tone. Respiratory arrest occurred repeatedly in the succeeding hours, and the infant died in 12 hours despite all measures to save her.

Histopathologic Examination. The ovarian cortical stroma is run through by relatively thick cords of primitive cells and a number of oogonia. More frequently the primitive cells form masses instead of cords (H & E, 375 ×).

At autopsy, in addition to generalized signs of immaturity, interatrial and interventricular septal defects were found. There were subtentorial and intraventricular hemorrhages as well as pulmonary anectasia and congenital pneumonia.

325
FOLLICULAR CYST OF OVARY

Female weighing 3,500 gm, 38 week gestational age. Apgar score 4 at birth. Generalized cyanosis, serious respiratory impairment, marked loss of tone and absence of spontaneous movements. On examination, imperforate anus and hypermobility of hip joints were noted. In spite of intensive therapeutic measures, the respiratory picture became worse, and the child died 2 hours after admission.

Histopathologic Examination. The internal genitalia included double vagina and double body of the uterus. There were two tubes and two ovaries with cysts. Figure 325 shows a large cyst lined by follicular epithelium with several Call-Exner bodies. The cyst cavity contains weakly staining fluid (H & E, 187.5 ×).

Autopsy showed the presence of pulmonary hypoplasia and intraalveolar hemorrhages. Marked distention of the entire colon and the upper part of the rectum was obvious. The latter terminated in a fibrous cord. There was a rectovesical fistula.

326/327
MESONEPHRIC REMNANTS IN THE OVARY

Full-term female weighing 3,150 gm. Admitted at 20 days of life because of serious diarrhea. On admission the infant was in poor general condition with signs of marked dehydration. Metabolic acidosis. Urine and blood cultures negative. Cultures of feces and nasal exudate positive for *Klebsiella*.

Chest x-rays showed scattered foci of bronchopneumonia. Urine was positive for albumin. In spite of rehydration, correction of acid-base imbalance, and antibiotic treatment, she died 12 days later.

Histopathologic Examination. The cortical zone of the ovary is thin and shows few follicles (Fig. 326, H & E, 60 ×). Deeper, within the medulla, there is an anomalous mass of tissue that, with greater magnification, is seen to contain tubular and glomeruloid structures; each of the latter is covered by a layer of tall epithelial cells (Fig. 327, H & E, 375 ×).

Other autopsy findings: Necrotizing enteritis and diffuse bronchopneumonia.

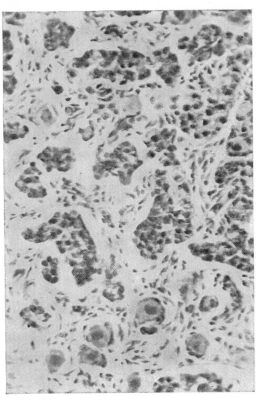

324

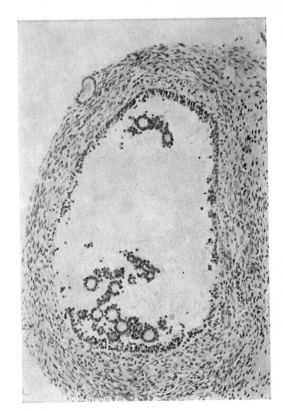

325

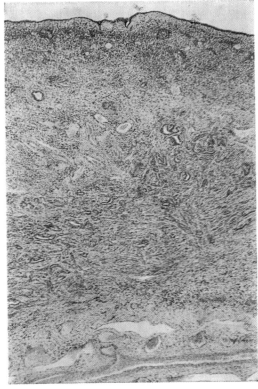

326

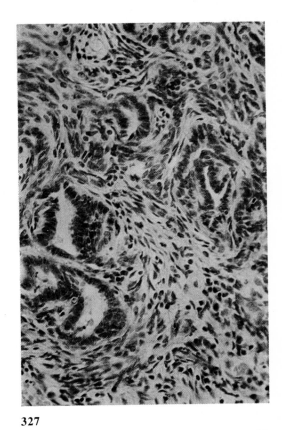

327

328
GRANULOMATOUS OOPHORITIS IN SEPSIS

Twenty-five day old female, weighing 3,400 gm, with no significant neonatal history. Admitted at this time because of severe diarrhea. Feedings had consisted of hyperconcentrated powdered milk. On examination, there were marked abdominal distention, poor general condition, and hypertonic dehydration. Chest x-ray showed infiltrative density in the right upper lung field. A diagnosis of generalized sepsis was considered. Blood culture was positive for *E. coli*. In spite of intensive therapeutic measures, she died 36 hours after admission.

Histopathologic Examination. Figure 328 shows granulomatous foci made up of some granulocytes and many monocytic cells within the medulla of the ovary (H & E, 60 ×).

Other autopsy findings included small granulomas in the myocardium.

329
CYTOMEGALIC INCLUSION DISEASE IN THE OVARY

Female weighing 1,150 gm, 29 week gestational age. Admitted at 2 hours of age with signs of immaturity, generalized loss of tone, and respiratory distress. Bouts of respiratory arrest necessitated repeated resuscitation. At 5 days, diarrhea and metabolic acidosis supervened. Three days later there was jaundice with total bilirubin of 10.5 mg/100 ml. The abdomen became distended, and the liver was palpable 2 fingerbreadths below the costal margin.

Culture of feces was positive for pathogenic *E. coli* type 0:86/B7. Subsequently the infant's general condition deteriorated. Direct bilirubin value was found to be 6.55 mg/100 ml, SGOT 425 u/L, SGPT 362 u/L. Blood culture was negative. A diagnosis of septic hepatitis was made. The child's condition deteriorated; jaundice persisted, and respiratory insufficiency appeared, accompanied by respiratory acidosis. pH 6.75, pCO$_2$ 70 mm Hg. Chest x-ray revealed bronchopneumonia.

Multiple examinations of urine sediment for cytomegalic cells were negative. She died 20 days after admission.

Histopathologic Examination. Figure 329 shows a number of cytomegalic cells with inclusions within the cortical zone of the ovary (H & E, 375 ×).

At autopsy there were similar cells in the liver, pancreas, and kidney.

330
PSEUDOPAPILLARY GLANDULAR HYPERPLASIA OF THE ENDOMETRIUM

Four day old female weighing 2,750 gm; gestational age, 38 weeks. Admitted for moderate perioral cyanosis and acrocyanosis. Femoral pulses were normal. Blood sugar, 78 mg/100 ml.

Two days later she suddenly developed the picture of cardiac failure, and a systolic murmur appeared in the right paratracheal area. A provisional diagnosis of congenital heart disease and transposition of the great arteries with interventricular septal defect or truncus arteriosus communis was made. Signs of cardiac failure subsided initially, but 9 days later frank decompensation was followed by death.

Histopathologic Examination. Figure 330 shows the endometrial lining of the corpus. The glands are overdeveloped and partially pseudopapillary (the uterine cavity was filled with mucinous material) (H & E, 60 ×).

At autopsy there was congenital heart disease and type I truncus arteriosus accompanied by signs of marked anoxia.

331
NEONATAL MASTITIS

Female weighing 1,950 gm; 41 weeks' gestational age; born by cesarean section. Admitted at 2 hours of life in poor general condition and with respiratory distress. A systolic murmur was audible in all valvular areas; the liver was enlarged to 2 fingerbreadths below the ribs, and there were several malformations of the face together with microcephaly. Chest x-ray showed cardiac enlargement with slight elevation of the apex; pulmonary vascularization was normal. Skull roentgenograms confirmed the presence of microcephaly with open sutures.

Death occurred at 24 hours after admission. Karyotyping revealed no numerical or structural chromosomal abnormalities. There was obvious mammary swelling.

Histopathologic Examination. The mammary stroma showed considerable inflammatory infiltration, predominantly by round cells, with scattered granulocytes. There was no abscess formation. The infiltrate is arranged around glandular elements. The latter contain a limited amount of secretion (H & E, 187.5 ×).

Autopsy showed multiple other anomalies.

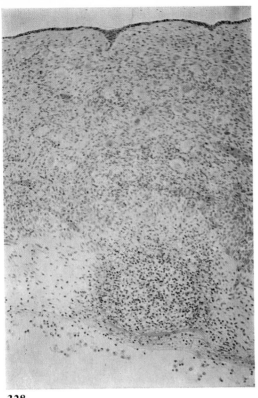

328

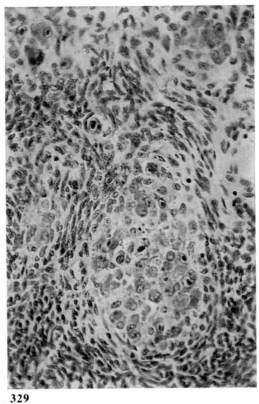

329

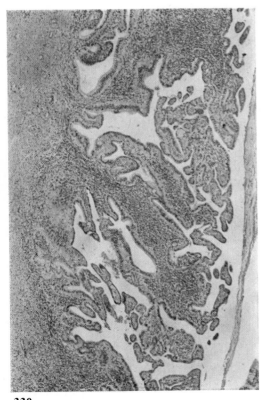

330

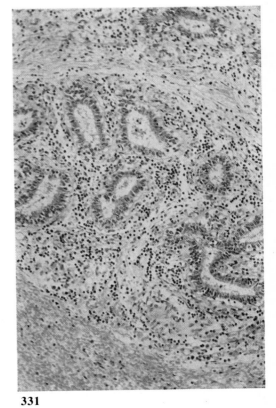

331

332
CYST OF THE CANAL OF NUCK

Fifteen day old female weighing 3,000 gm, born at term. Admitted because of the presence of a small mass in the left inguinal region. The lesion was the size of a hazelnut and could not be reduced into the abdomen manually. The rest of the physical examination was normal. Surgical intervention revealed a left inguinal hernia and a cyst of the canal of Nuck. The postoperative course was uneventful.

Histopathologic Examination. The cavity of the cystic mass is lined by a single layer of flattened epithelial cells. The wall consists of loose connective tissue. There are perivascular inflammatory infiltrates made up of round cells (187.5 ×).

333
ANEMIC INFARCT OF THE TESTICLE

Male, born at term, weighing 4,600 gm. At birth a hard mass was detected, firmly attached to the left testicle. At 21 days of age the infant was admitted because of persistent crying and an increase in size of the mass, which was adherent to the scrotum; it was tender and accompanied by marked scrotal cyanosis. Immediate surgical exploration demonstrated torsion of the testicle and the terminal portion of the spermatic cord. The testicle was completely necrotic, the tunica vaginalis was thickened, and there was a blood-tinged hydrocele. It was deemed necessary to remove the testicle. Postoperative course was normal.

Histopathologic Examination. Figure 333 shows extensive coagulation necrosis of the tubules, which are represented by "shadow" images; there is no interstitial hemorrhage nor is there hemosiderin pigment. At the lower end of the figure there is a group of partly preserved tubules (H & E, 187.5 ×).

334
INTERSTITIAL HEMORRHAGE OF THE TESTICLE

Male weighing 3,000 gm, 37 weeks' gestational age. Admitted 1 hour after birth, with irregular respiration and severe cyanosis. The fontanelles were widened; there was bilateral pes varus, and each hand showed an accessory digit next to the thumb. Metabolic acidosis. Shortly thereafter the respiratory insufficiency increased, and he expelled bloody mucus by mouth and nose. At 8 hours of life the infant expired. Karyotyping had not shown numerical or structural anomalies.

Histopathologic Examination. Interstitial hemorrhage of the testicle is a frequent finding in newborns dying in anoxia (Translators' note: and those delivered by breech extraction.)

Figure 334 shows massive interstitial hemorrhage. The seminiferous tubules are preserved; the lining cells are intact (H & E, 60 ×). Compare with Figure 335.

In addition to the aforementioned anomalies, autopsy showed an ossification defect of the skull with ample communication between the two fontanelles, abundant subarachnoid hemorrhage, massive left-sided pulmonary hemorrhage, cutaneous petechiae, and microcystic renal changes.

335
HEMORRHAGIC INFARCT OF TESTICLE

Male weighing 3,000 gm; gestational age, 40 weeks. Admitted at 3 hours of life. Apgar score 7 at birth. Moribund on admission, with hypothermia, marked pallor of skin and mucosae, moderate jaundice, generalized edema, bradycardia, moderate dyspnea, serious loss of muscle tone, and bulging abdomen with marked hepatosplenomegaly. The mother's blood was group B, Rh (D) negative.

The newborn's blood was group O, Rh (D) positive with positive direct Coombs reaction. Total bilirubin 8.2 mg/100 ml, microhematocrit 16 per cent, pH 6.95, total protein 3.0 mg/100 ml. Immediately on admission, hypertonic glucose, digitalis, and bicarbonate were administered, followed by exchange transfusion with packed red cells. Death occurred 4 hours after admission, in the midst of treatment.

Histopathologic Examination. The left testicle showed marked hemorrhagic infiltration. In contrast with Figure 334, the seminiferous tubules are necrotic and remain only as shadows with faint basophilic staining (H & E, 187.5 ×).

In general, the autopsy findings were consistent with those of erythroblastosis fetalis with marked extramedullary hematopoiesis. There were also aspiration of meconium and petechial hemorrhages in the pleura, lung, pericardium, adrenals, and brain.

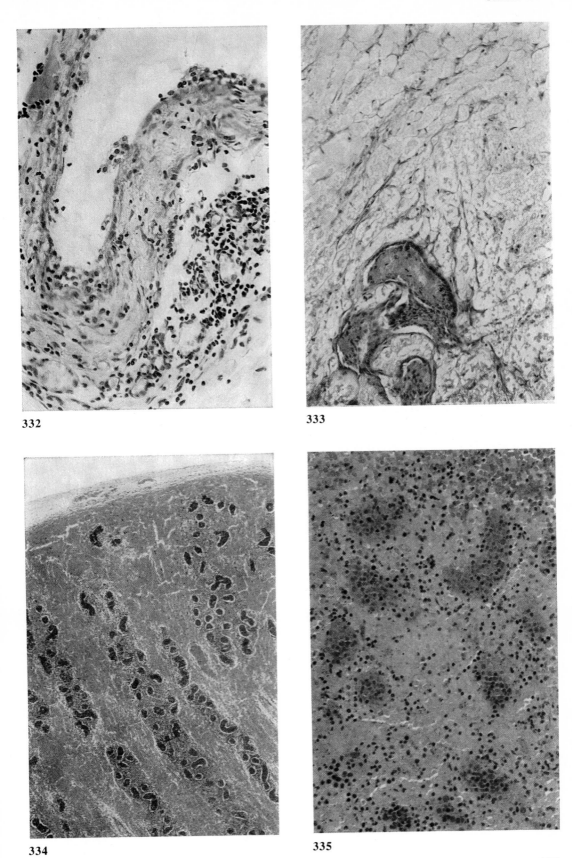

332

333

334

335

336
IMMATURE TESTICLE

Male weighing 770 gm; gestational age, 21 weeks. Apgar score 1 at birth. Moderate respiratory distress, bradycardia, areflexia, and severe hypotonicity. Dead on arrival at pediatric intensive care unit.

Histopathologic Examination. The seminiferous tubules show a lining of primitive cells with a number of rounded and acidophilic spermatogonia (H & E, 375 ×).

Note the presence in the interstitium of eosinophilic Leydig cells. Such cells usually disappear in full-term infants. The autopsy disclosed signs of generalized immaturity as well as congenital pneumonia.

337
LEYDIG CELL HYPERPLASIA

Male weighing 2,650 gm. Gestational age, 35 weeks. Vertex delivery; Apgar score 9 at birth. Four hours later, signs of respiratory distress appeared, necessitating admission. Examination showed cyanosis, rapid breathing, and edema of eyelids. pH 7.07, pCO_2 89 mm Hg, BE −7.5 mEq/L. Chest x-ray showed a large thymus and an image compatible with grade II pulmonary hyaline membrane disease. Despite treatment, the child's clinical course was downhill, and he died at 48 hours of age.

Histopathologic Examination. The seminiferous tubules are immature and consist primarily of undifferentiated germinal cells and occasional spermatogonia. There is a striking number of eosinophilic Leydig cells, which occupy virtually the entire interstitial space (H & E, 375 ×).

Necropsy showed pulmonary atelectasis and abundant pulmonary hyaline membranes with clusters of granulocytes in some air spaces. Signs of immaturity were especially obvious in the kidney and liver.

338/339
NODULAR HYPERPLASIA OF LEYDIG CELLS

Male weighing 2,300 gm at 34 weeks' gestational age, admitted 30 minutes after birth. Apgar score 5 at birth, requiring resuscitation, intubation, and assisted respiration. Very poor condition on admission, slow heart beat, marked hepatomegaly, and peripheral edema. Mixed acidosis.

Rh isoimmunization was diagnosed. He died 3 hours later in respiratory insufficiency. Chest x-ray had shown right-sided pneumothorax.

Histopathologic Examination. It is not uncommon to encounter Leydig cell hyperplasia in the testicle of a premature infant. Figure 338 shows nodular adenomatoid hyperplasia of interstitial cells (H & E, 60 ×).

With greater magnification, the acidophilic character of the cytoplasm of these cells can be observed, as well as the arrangement in well-delimited micronodules (Fig. 339, H & E, 187.5 ×).

At autopsy, considerable hematopoietic activity was noted in the liver. The right lung showed atelectasis and anectasia with pneumothorax. There was hemorrhage in the glandular portion of the pituitary and in the islets of Langerhans. The adrenals showed some cytomegaly. Signs of immaturity were evident throughout.

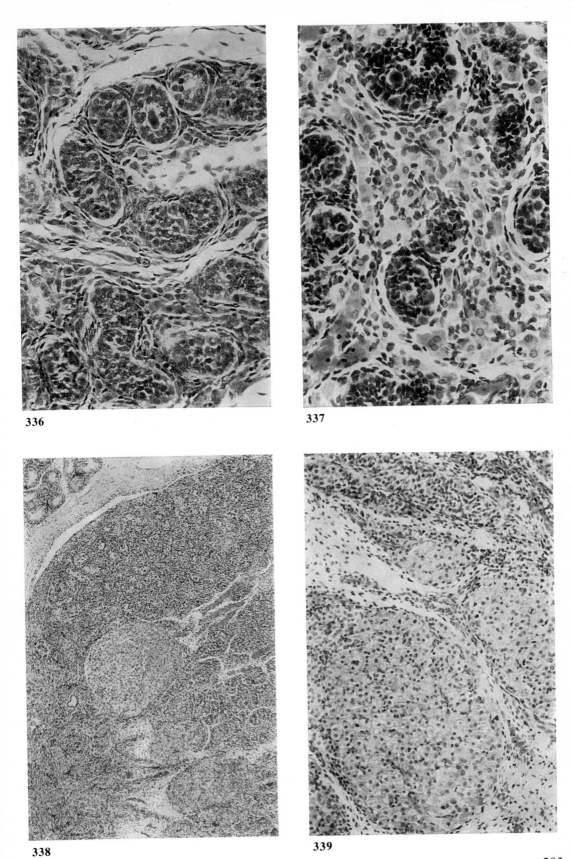

336

337

338

339

Lymphatic System

340
THYMUS WITH "STARRY-SKY" PATTERN

Male weighing 1600 gm. Gestational age, 32 weeks, twin birth. Difficult delivery with Apgar score 3 at birth necessitating energetic resuscitation. Admitted 2 days after birth in poor general condition with marked loss of tone, jaundice, and dehydration. On admission, total bilirubin was 18.4 mg/100 ml, hematocrit 42 per cent, total protein 4.7 gm/100 ml, pH 7.09, pCO_2 71 mm Hg, BE −11.5 mEq/L. Clinical picture of sepsis. X-ray of the chest was normal. Blood culture, negative. Stool culture, negative for *Salmonella* and enteropathogenic *E. coli;* few colonies of *Candida*. Culture of pharyngeal exudate showed numerous colonies of *E. coli* and *Aerobacter aerogenes*. Spinal fluid culture, negative. Urine culture, 230,000 colonies of *Klebsiella* per milliliter of cultured urine. General condition became progressively worse. The infant died at 13 days of life with abdominal distention and diarrhea.

Histopathologic Examination. The lymphocytic population of the cortical zone of the thymus is within normal limits and contrasts with the lighter-staining medullary zone. In the midst of the cortical area there are numerous scattered reticulum cells with light-staining cytoplasm, creating the so-called "starry-sky" pattern. Autopsy revealed necrotizing enteritis with pneumatosis cystoides intestinalis.

341
INVERSION OF THYMIC ARCHITECTURAL PATTERN

Male weighing 1,340 gm. Gestational age, 30 weeks. Admitted 1 hour after birth in poor general condition with cyanosis and edema. pH 7.25, pCO_2 51 mm Hg, BE −6 mEq/L. From the second day on, the infant experienced repeated bouts of apnea and hypertonic episodes. Bloody spinal fluid was negative on culture. Blood culture was similarly negative, but cultures of gastric contents and meconium produced colonies of *E. coli* and *Klebsiella*. He had marked hypothermia, and his respiratory insufficiency became worse. Chest x-ray was diagnosed as pneumonia. He died at 5 days.

Histopathologic Examination. Figure 341 shows a light-staining cortical area produced by marked depletion of lymphocytes with apparent reticulum cell hyperplasia. This produces a seeming inversion of the normal pattern in which the cortical zone is more darkly stained because of its greater lymphocytic density. Hassall's corpuscles are relatively prominent here, again because of lymphocytic depletion.

At autopsy there was necrotizing bronchopneumonia with subarachnoid and periventricular hemorrhage.

342
CALCIFICATION OF HASSALL'S CORPUSCLES

Female weighing 2,880 gm. Gestational age, 41 weeks. Admitted 15 hours after birth because of multiple malformations corresponding clinically to trisomy 13. This diagnosis was confirmed by study of the peripheral karyotype. At the same time there was respiratory difficulty and metabolic acidosis. There was a 2–3/6 midsystolic murmur, heard best over the precordium. Later, x-ray of the chest showed bronchopneumonia. She died at 16 days.

Histopathologic Examination. The thymus was atrophic, weighing only 4 gm, and showed apparent enlargement and calcification of the majority of Hassall's corpuscles.

In addition, autopsy showed osseous malformations affecting the calcification centers, agenesis of the olfactory bulbs and tracts, islands of aberrant cerebellar tissue, and atrioventricularis communis. There was bronchopneumonia with aspiration of amniotic debris.

343
SECONDARY ATROPHY OF THYMUS

Male weighing 1,340 gm. Gestational age, 30 weeks. Admitted 1 hour after birth with signs of marked immaturity, cyanosis, and edema of the lower extremities. With standard treatment the infant's course was uneventful until the third day of life. From that time on there were multiple episodes of hypertonicity. Spinal tap yielded hemorrhagic fluid. Culture of the fluid was negative. The picture of respiratory insufficiency became worse. X-ray of the chest showed signs of bronchopneumonia and aspiration. Culture of meconium and gastric contents yielded multiple colonies of *E. coli* and *Klebsiella*. Antibiotics were administered. Hypertonicity increased and also respiratory insufficiency, leading to death at 11 days of life.

Histopathologic Examination. The thymus was markedly atrophic, weighing 3 gm, with considerable predominance of the connective tissue stroma. There was marked lymphoid depletion and practically complete absence of the cortical zone. Hassall's corpuscles were prominent.

Autopsy showed subarachnoid and intraventricular hemorrhages.

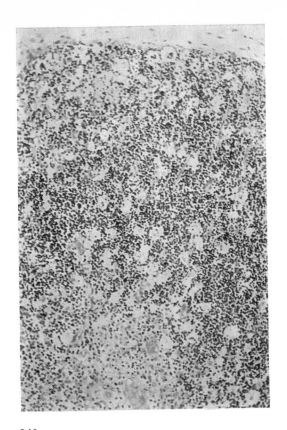

340

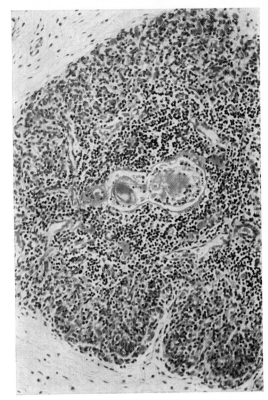

341

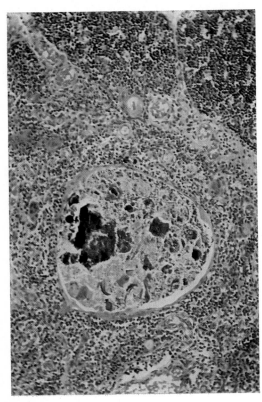

342

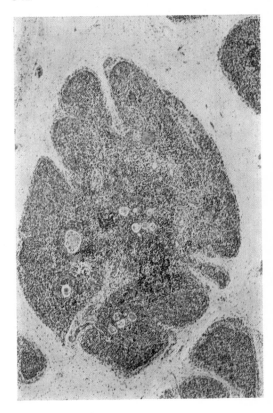

343

344/345
DiGEORGE SYNDROME

Male weighing 3,440 gm. Gestational age, 40 weeks. Apgar score 2 at birth, necessitating intensive resuscitation. Admitted 3 hours later. On admission the general appearance was poor, with generalized cyanosis, plaintive cry, shallow respirations, and hepatomegaly. Cardiac auscultation showed splitting of the first heart sound in both the tricuspid and pulmonary areas. Chest x-ray showed a globular heart shadow. The infant was placed in an incubator with oxygen and in the next few hours had repeated episodes of respiratory arrest. Treatment for cardiac insufficiency was to no avail. Death occurred 10 hours after birth.

Histopathologic Examination. At autopsy there was no thymus, and serial microscopic sections of the anterior cervical region did not reveal any thymic remnants nor any parathyroids.

Figure 344 shows a mesenteric lymph node with a markedly thin cortical zone, with dilated medullary sinusoids and narrow and depleted medullary cords. (For comparison, Figure 345 represents a lymph node from a child of the same age and weight.) This image is observed in reactive lymph nodes in a more advanced stage of life, in which follicular hyperplasia stands out as against the absence of any response of the paracortical thymic dependent zone.

At autopsy there were no significant external anomalies. There was generalized visceral congestion, pulmonary atelectasis, and congenital atresia of the pulmonary valve together with interatrial and interventricular septal defects, persistence of the ductus arteriosus, and hypertrophy of the right ventricle.

346
IMMATURE LYMPH NODE REACTION

Female weighing 3,600 gm. Gestational age, 42 weeks. Admitted at 8 days of life with respiratory difficulty. On examination there was poor general condition, bilateral cephalhematoma, and 1 fingerbreadth hepatosplenomegaly. Mixed acidosis. pO_2 in 50 per cent oxygen, 81 mm Hg. Chest x-ray showed bilateral coarse areas of consolidation, confluent in places. Cultures of blood, urine, spinal fluid, and stool were negative. Cultures of gastric contents and pharyngeal exudate yielded colonies of *Klebsiella* and *Enterobacter*. During the hours following admission her general condition deteriorated. Respiratory insufficiency worsened, necessitating intubation and assisted respiration, and the infant died 15 hours after admission with the clinical diagnosis of bronchopneumonia.

Histopathologic Examination. Figure 346 shows the cortical zone of a mesenteric lymph node. The subcapsular sinus is dilated and filled with granulocytes and histiocytes. A similar picture is found in the medullary sinusoids. Note the absence of reactive follicles. The presence of macrophages with light-staining cytoplasm scattered in the diffuse portion of the cortex creates a sort of "starry sky" image. There was no paracortical reaction.

At autopsy there were large areas of confluent bronchopneumonia in both lungs, general signs of sepsis, and hyaline thrombi in the capillaries of the liver and the adrenals, with visceral petechiae suggesting generalized intravascular coagulation.

347
PARACORTICAL LYMPHOID HYPERPLASIA

Male weighing 2,170 gm. Gestational age unknown. Admitted at 12 days of life with severe respiratory insufficiency. There was atresia of the esophagus that had been diagnosed the previous day. X-ray examination confirmed the presence of atresia of the esophagus with tracheoesophageal fistula, bilateral bronchopneumonia, and considerable atelectasis in the right lung field. Mixed metabolic and respiratory acidosis. pO_2 in 50 per cent oxygen, 70 mm Hg. Parenteral alimentation was started. Three days later the tracheoesophageal fistula was ligated and end-to-end anastomosis of the esophagus was accomplished. During the ensuing days respiratory insufficiency became worse. The patient's general condition worsened, and x-ray of the chest showed extension of the bronchopneumonia. Death occured 3 days after surgery. Cultures of the pharynx on admission yielded *E. coli*.

Histopathologic Examination. The pulmonary hilar lymph nodes showed no reactive follicles. The cortical zone was thickened by an increase in the paracortical and interfollicular components with prominent postcapillary venules. There were many blast cells (large lymphocytes), as shown in Figure 347. The sinusoids were dilated and filled with macrophages. This image corresponds to a thymic dependent reaction and suggests, although it is not diagnostic of, a viral infection. The lung showed a desquamative necrotizing pneumonia with moderate septal infiltration by round cells, a picture similar to that seen in Figures 44 and 45. There were no inclusion bodies.

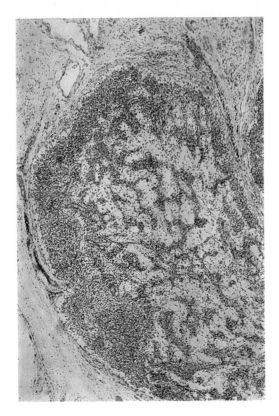

344

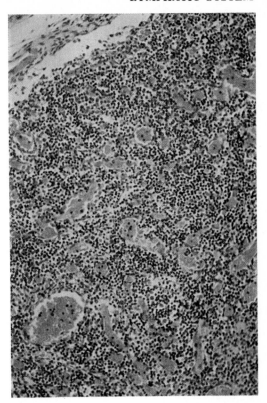

345

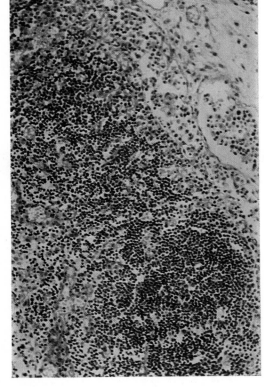

346

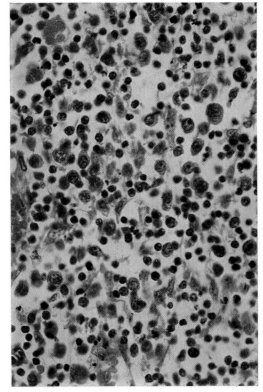

347

CYSTOID LYMPHADENITIS

Female weighing 1,960 gm. Gestational age, 40 weeks. Mother had had a white vaginal discharge during this pregnancy. The infant was admitted 3 days after delivery in poor general condition with hypotonia and probable hepatosplenomegaly. Jaundice with 15.23 mg/100 ml total bilirubin. Microhematocrit 44 per cent, 15,400 leukocytes per cubic millimeter. Diarrhea. Metabolic acidosis. Blood culture was positive for *Klebsiella*. The patient's diarrhea and poor general condition persisted. She died on the eighth day of life.

Histopathologic Examination. Mesenteric lymph nodes: The sinusoids of the node are markedly dilated, with the formation of cystic cavities that lend the node a multilocular appearance. There is no giant cell reaction such as occurs in the cystoid adenitis produced by the injection of contrast media in the conduct of a lymphangiogram.

Autopsy showed acute enteritis with pneumatosis cystoides intestinalis and fibrinous peritonitis. There was also a subcapsular hematoma of the liver.

349/350
CONGENITAL RUBELLA SECONDARY FOLLICLES

Male weighing 2,300 gm. Gestational age, 40 weeks. Apgar score 9 at birth. Admitted 15 minutes after delivery with signs of dysmaturity, dry and fissured skin, patches of brownish discoloration of the skin 1 to 5 mm in diameter scattered over the entire body, and hepatosplenomegaly. After a few hours respiratory difficulty appeared and a systolic murmur could be heard. A chest x-ray showed the presence of total cardiac enlargement with increase in pulmonary circulation and normal pulmonary parenchyma. Serologic tests were negative, as were cultures of blood, urine, meconium, and spinal fluid. Hematocrit 67 per cent, hemoglobin 15 gm/100 ml, platelets 20,000/cu mm. Normal ophthalmologic examination.

X-rays of the skeleton showed radiolucent bands at the metaphyses of the long bones. Both distal femoral metaphyses showed very irregular proximal edges with radiolucent striations parallel to the axis of the shaft. The spinal column, pelvis, and cranial vault were radiographically normal. The bone lesions and splenomegaly suggested the diagnosis of intrauterine viral infection. The association of these anomalies with cardiomegaly and pulmonary hyperemia pointed to the probable presence of a congenital cardiac anomaly with a left-to-right shunt, supporting the diagnosis of congenital rubella infection. Although there was no history of maternal rubella infection in the early months of gestation, there had been a significant outbreak of rubella at that time in the city where the mother lived.

Test for antibody titer by means of hemagglutination inhibition was positive at 1:64 in the infant. IgM on the third day of life was 78 mg/100 ml. Cardiac insufficiency ensued, and in spite of treatment the infant died at 4 days of age.

Histopathologic Examination. Figure 349 shows a malpighian corpuscle in the spleen. Note its reactive appearance with central accumulation of epithelioid cells, scattered macrophages, and abundant nuclear remnants. Large lymphocytes are predominant at the periphery of the follicle. The lymph nodes also show cortical secondary follicles, an anomalous finding, considering the age of the infant, as well as marked hyperplasia of the paracortical zone (Fig. 350).

Other autopsy findings included a widely patent ductus arteriosus, subarachnoid and intracerebral hemorrhage, pulmonary edema and hemorrhage, and changes in the hepatic architecture with portal fibrosis and alterations in the columns of liver cells.

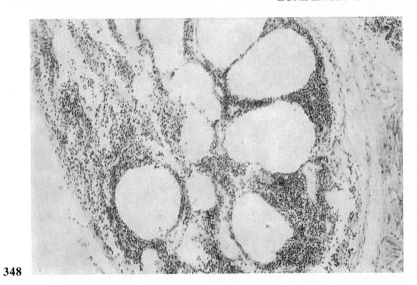

348

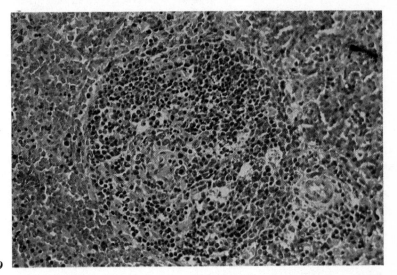

349

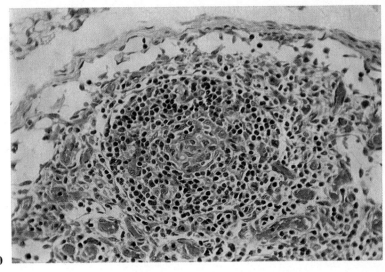

350

EXTRAMEDULLARY HEMATOPOIESIS IN SPLEEN AND LYMPH NODES

Male weighing 3,300 gm. Gestational age, 40 weeks. At delivery, amniotic fluid was tinted with meconium. The infant had a weak cry, respiratory difficulty, and jaundice. Admitted at 6 hours of age in poor general condition. Cardiorespiratory arrest responded to cardiac massage and assisted respiration with intubation. There was hepatosplenomegaly and jaundice, with generalized loss of tone. Metabolic acidosis. X-ray of the chest showed disseminated areas of consolidation in both lung fields with obvious air bronchogram. Hematocrit 26 per cent. Total bilirubin 10 mg/100 ml. Blood type O Rh (D) positive. Direct Coombs test, positive. The mother was O Rh (D) negative. Cardiac arrest occurred 2 hours after admission before an exchange transfusion could be attempted.

Histopathologic Examination. The spleen weighed 29 gm and showed marked extramedullary hematopoiesis, with effacement of the normal architecture of the organ. Sinusoidal macrophages were loaded with hemosiderin (Fig. 351). Lymph nodes also showed foci of hematopoiesis, especially in the pericapsular connective tissue (Fig. 352).

Other autopsy findings included the presence of hepatomegaly, moderate cardiac enlargement, and hyperplasia of the adrenals. Microscopically, there was hyperplasia of pancreatic islets, and there were hematopoietic foci in various other organs.

In erythroblastosis, extramedullary hematopoiesis compensates for the hemolysis of isoimmunity, especially that of Rh incompatibility, and it represents either an exaggeration or an anomalous prolongation of the extramedullary hematopoiesis that is normal during fetal life. Another important cause of extramedullary hematopoiesis in the neonatal period, especially in prematures, is infection in which marked proliferation of myeloid cells in extramedullary sites can be observed. This is particularly notable in the portal areas of the liver. It probably represents stimulation of the pluripotential mesenchymal cells and their return to a phase of activity similar to that of the fetal period. In cytomegalic inclusion disease and in toxoplasmosis the extramedullary response is predominantly erythroblastic. In all of these infections there are usually many eosinophils in the foci of hematopoiesis.

353
CONGENITAL LEUKEMIA. SPLENIC INVOLVEMENT

Female weighing 2,680 gm. Gestational age, 41 weeks. Vertex presentation at delivery. Apgar score 10 at 1 minute. Admitted 1 hour after delivery in good general condition. There were many brown maculopapular lesions, measuring about 3 cm in diameter, diffusely scattered over the body and scalp. Normal chest x-ray. Peripheral blood showed: leukocytes 5,300/cu mm (eosinophils 0, stab cells 1, segmented 20, lymphocytes 57, monocytes 6, and blasts 16 per cent). Platelets 90,000/cu mm. Biopsy of the skin showed that in the dermis and deep subcutaneous tissue there were numerous groups of atypical cells with relatively large and irregular nuclei and scanty cytoplasm. There were no metachromatic granules in the cytoplasm of the neoplastic cells. This picture corresponds to that of a malignant infiltrative process, either a malignant form of reticuloendotheliosis or blast cell leukemia. Bone marrow examination showed: erythroblasts 24.5, myeloblasts 2, promyelocytes 19.5, myelocytes 27, metamyelocytes 8.5, band forms 7.5, segmented 6.5, lymphocytes 3, and reticuloendothelial cells 1.5 per cent respectively. The myelocytes, promyelocytes, and myeloblasts were giant irregular cells with cytoplasmic vacuoles and scanty granulations. The entire bone marrow was hypocellular.

Decreased clot retraction, prothrombin 75 per cent, fibrinogen 1 gm/100 ml. Cephalin 57.5 seconds. Cultures of meconium, gastric contents, pharyngeal smear, and urine were negative. Serologic tests negative. Diagnosis of congenital promyelocytic leukemia was established. In spite of adequate treatment she developed buccal thrush, diarrhea, respiratory insufficiency, leukopenia, and severe platelet deficiency with a hemorrhagic syndrome.

Later cultures of gastric contents and pharyngeal smear were positive for *E. coli,* and in the stool culture *Candida* was isolated. The child died 21 days after admission.

Histopathologic Examination. Figure 353 shows a section of spleen with leukemic infiltration limited to the walls of the trabecular vessels. There was marked lymphoid depletion, which was also present in the thymus and lymph nodes. This type of infiltration of walls of blood vessels is seen often in the acute leukemias of infancy. (In erythroblastosis fetalis, foci of hematopoiesis may be seen in the walls of blood vessels.) In addition to leukemic infiltration of the bone marrow, autopsy showed hemorrhagic gastritis and necrotizing enterocolitis.

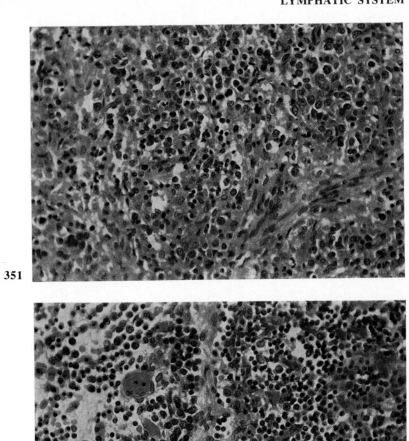

351

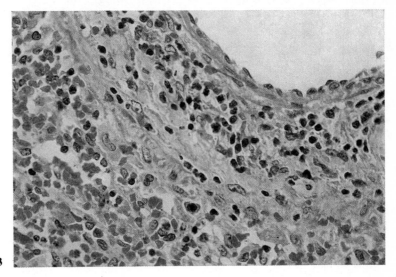

352

353

The Eye

354
ANOPHTHALMIA

Male weighing 2,300 gm. Gestational age unknown. Admitted 2 hours after birth because of congenital anomalies including anophthalmia, bilateral clubfeet, pigeon breast, and low implantation of the ears. The presence of a rectal membrane 3 cm above the anal opening was demonstrated by x-ray and by digital examination. It was incised, whereupon meconium poured out freely. X-ray of the skull showed no intracranial calcifications or any other malformations. The configuration of the orbital cavity was normal. EEG showed a normal pattern in keeping with the age of the subject. Karyotype showed a 44 XY pattern with no anomalies.

In the days following admission, there were respiratory signs attributable to minimal aspiration of amniotic debris. Development was deficient. The weight held steady, but the infant died 25 days later of bronchopneumonia.

Histopathologic Examination. Orbital cavities: The only presumably ocular structures found were represented by vascular tissue with numerous pigmented cells and calcific remnants (H & E, 375 ×).

At autopsy there was moderate microgyria. The optic chiasm and optic nerves were present. There were four accessory spleens in the area of the gastrosplenic ligament. There were microcysts in the kidneys. Death was attributed to pulmonary cytomegalic disease and excessive aspiration of amniotic debris.

355
RETINAL DYSPLASIA WITH PERSISTENT PRIMARY VITREOUS

Male weighing 1,050 gm. Gestational age, 28 weeks. Twin pregnancy. Apgar score 8 at birth. Admitted 2 hours after delivery in poor general condition with marked loss of tone, cyanosis, and general signs of immaturity. pH 7.19, pCO_2 55 mm Hg, BE −9 mEq/L. Microhematocrit 62 per cent. Total protein 3.9 gm/100 ml. Acidosis was treated with intravenous dextrose and bicarbonate, and the infant was placed in an incubator. One hour later apneic episodes intervened, with marked deterioration of the infant's general condition and a cardiac arrest, which was converted. The apneic episodes recurred in the following 2 hours, and death occurred 13 hours after birth. Blood culture was negative.

Histopathologic Examination. Figure 355 shows the posterior chamber of the globe. It seems to be filled with connective tissue with many vascular areas such as can be seen in the lower part of the illustration and a few clusters of fat cells. There are also partly tubular retinal anlagen, indicating the dysplastic nature of the lesion (H & E, 60 ×).

At autopsy there was pulmonary immaturity. Petechiae were found in the thymus and epicardium. There were foci of necrosis in the myocardium and bilateral intraventricular hemorrhages as well as microophthalmia.

356/357
TOXOPLASMA CHORIORETINITIS

Female weighing 2,480 gm. Gestational age, 32 weeks. The same case as is illustrated in Figures 116, 156/157, and 317.

Histopathologic Examination. The retina and the choroid show multiple changes, especially granulation tissue with newly formed capillaries and abundant round cell infiltration. In the center there is a cleft with a pigmented uveal remnant (Fig. 356, H & E, 375 ×).

With higher magnification, in the midst of this tissue, cysts of *Toxoplasma* appear as amphophilic spherules containing small basophilic bodies (Fig. 357, H & E, 600 ×).

At autopsy there was internal hydrocephalus with necrotic and granulomatous foci in the brain (Figs. 156 and 157), myocardium (Fig. 116), and adrenal (Fig. 317, supporting the diagnosis of toxoplasmosis.

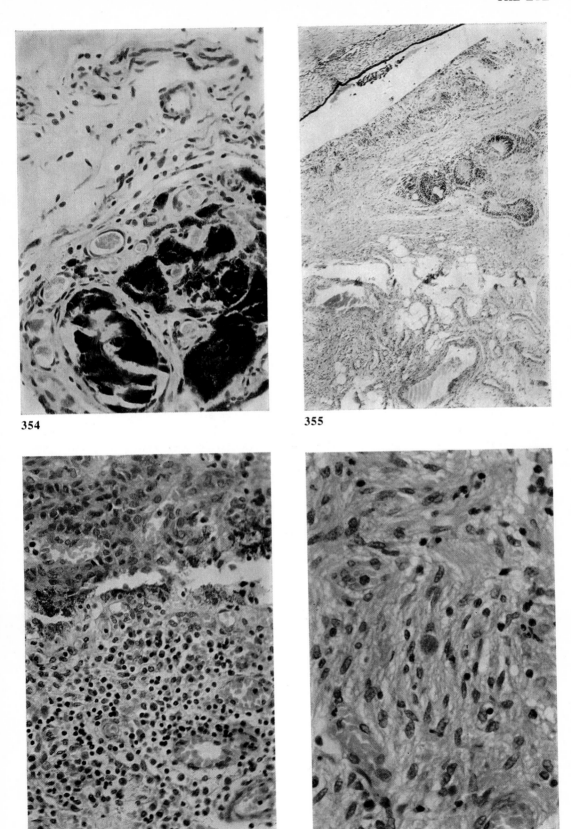

354

355

356

357

358/359
ADVANCED RETROLENTAL FIBROPLASIA

Male weighing 1,350 gm. Unknown gestational age. Twin birth. Admitted 4 hours after delivery in very poor general condition with marked cyanosis and considerable hypotonia. Chest x-ray showed a picture compatible with the diagnosis of pulmonary hyaline membrane disease. Mixed respiratory and metabolic acidosis was corrected with 10 per cent dextrose and 1 M bicarbonate infusion. Arterial pO_2 in 30 per cent oxygen atmosphere, 40 mm Hg, and in 100 per cent oxygen, 60 mm Hg. In the ensuing days there were repeated episodes of respiratory arrest requiring resuscitation and the administration of oxygen. The clinical course after that was good, and the child was released 65 days later weighing 2,530 gm and apparently normal except for retrolental fibroplasia.

Twenty days after being discharged he was again admitted with an acute respiratory process and what seemed to be hepatitis. Death occurred 2 days later. During this admission, ophthalmologic examination confirmed the presence of an advanced degree of retrolental fibroplasia.

Histopathologic Examination. The retina was detached, leaving a space filled with homogeneous acidophilic material. Note the scalloped appearance of the retinal tunic produced by the presence of connective tissue and vessels on its anterior aspect. The lens is displaced and does not appear in this preparation (Fig. 358, H & E, 15 ×).

With greater magnification, the very loose appearance of the sparsely cellular connective tissue can be seen, as well as vessels with considerable swelling of their walls. The retina shows a normal cellular architectural arrangement (Fig. 359, H & E, 187.5 ×).

At autopsy, giant cell hepatitis was demonstrated as well as bacterial bronchopneumonia.

360/361
RETINAL DYSPLASIA

Male weighing 3,000 gm. Gestational age, 40 weeks. Born by cesarean section. Apgar score 2 at birth, requiring intensive resuscitation. Admitted at 1 hour of age with cyanosis, deep depression, and a number of malformations including moderate microcephaly, microophthalmia, cleft palate with hare lip, hypoplastic penis, and congenital heart disease. Ophthalmologic examination showed no changes other than the bilateral microopthalmia.

Arterial pulse normal. Low pansystolic murmur with a split second sound, prolonged and constant. Hemoglobin saturation 74 per cent. X-ray examination showed moderate cardiac enlargement with a probable increase of pulmonary circulation. ECG revealed a right bundle branch block. There seemed to be right ventricular hypertrophy with probable diastolic overload. The general impression was of an interventricular septal defect with transposition of the great vessels or an anomalous pulmonary venous return. Study of the karyotype permitted establishment of the diagnosis of trisomy 13. The child died 15 days later with an acute inflammatory process and cardiac insufficiency.

Histopathologic Examination. Figure 360 shows a section of the eye with marked irregularity of the retinal architecture. It is also apparent, on the left side of the illustration, that there is a cartilaginous plaque (H & E, 15 ×).

Figure 361, at greater magnification, shows tubular retinal formations in various stages of development near the perichondrium of the plaque (H & E, 60 ×).

The autopsy also demonstrated bronchopneumonia, transposition of great vessels, interventricular septal defect, and hypoplasia of the left ventricle in addition to the already described anomalies.

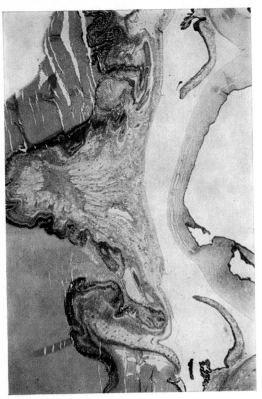

358

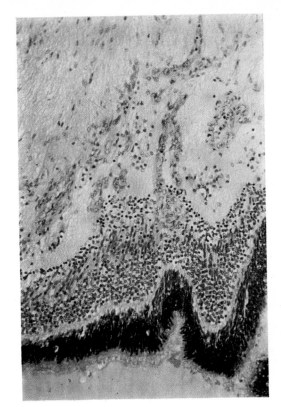

359

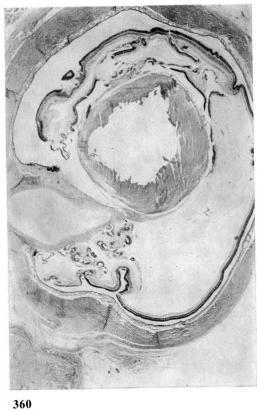

360

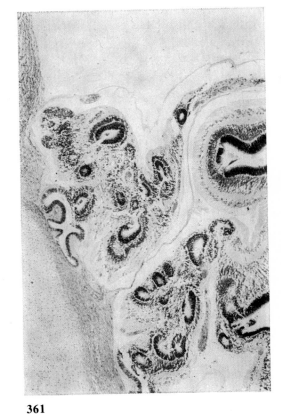

361

Skeletal System

362/363/364/365
OSTEOGENESIS IMPERFECTA

Female weighing 1,950 gm. Gestational age, 38 weeks. Apgar score at birth 7. Breech delivery. Admitted at 2 hours of age with cyanosis and in poor general condition; there was generalized hypotonia with diminished response to stimuli and a weak cry. Examination showed the presence of respiratory insufficiency with marked hypoventilation. On palpation, the head felt like celluloid and crackled. The cranial circumference was 31.5 cm, and the length of the body 36 cm. The extremities were short and curved, and gentle palpation of the bones elicited a crackling sensation. Acid-base study showed respiratory acidosis. Calcium, phosphorus, and phosphatase levels were within normal limits. A skeletal survey showed marked generalized rarefaction accompanied by multiple fractures compatible with the pattern of osteogenesis imperfecta. Death occurred at 12 hours of life.

Histopathologic Examination. Figure 362 shows a costochondral junction stained for alkaline phosphatase. There is enzyme activity in the area, and the cartilage appears normal (187.5 ×).

Figure 363 represents a preparation with reticulin stain that shows abnormality in the formation of spicular bone with remnants of cartilaginous matrix irregularly surrounded by silver-staining material (Wilder's stain, 375 ×).

Figure 364 shows the irregular appearance of a rib with numerous fractures and callus at different stages of development (H & E, 15 ×).

With greater magnification, one sees an old subperiostial fracture with irregular cartilaginous plates undergoing ossification. The bone marrow in the vicinity is fibrous and shows no hematopoiesis (Fig. 365, H & E, 60 ×).

Autopsy showed pulmonary hypoplasia and signs of anoxia with petechiae and visceral hemorrhages.

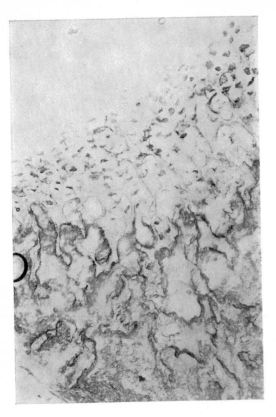

362

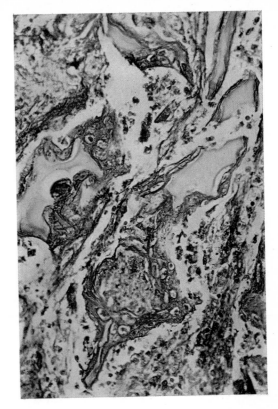

363

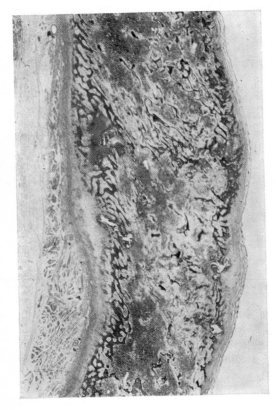

364

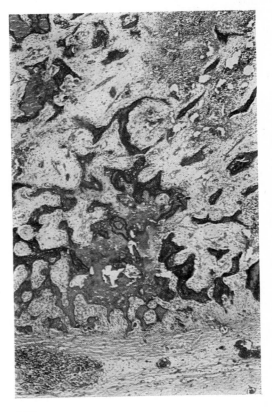

365

366
ACHONDROPLASIA (HYPOPLASTIC CHONDRODYSTROPHY)

Female weighing 3,760 gm. Gestational age, 38 weeks. Admitted 3 days after birth with respiratory insufficiency. Examination showed a large skull, "saddle" nose, bell-shaped thorax, and low-placed umbilicus. X-rays revealed a normal sized trunk with deformed vertebrae, particularly in the dorsolumbar region, marked lumbar lordosis, and a flattened pelvis. The bones of the extremities were foreshortened, with short diaphysis and widening of the epiphysis. The diagnosis of achondroplasia was made. Respiratory distress was attributed to bacterial pneumonia. The infant died 3 days later.

Histopathologic Examination. There was marked deformity of the costochondral junction. The cartilage cells form irregularly distributed, abnormally arranged rows. Vascular supply to the cartilage and bony trabecuale is also irregular. The bone marrow is essentially normal at this level (H & E, 187.5 ×).

At autopsy there were foci of bronchopneumonia accompanied by edema and pulmonary hemorrhage. The foramen magnum was deformed by cartilaginous masses.

367/368
ALBERS-SCHÖNBERG DISEASE (OSTEOPETROSIS)

Female weighing 3,250 gm, born at 42 weeks' gestational age. Admitted at 15 days of life because of left-sided faciobrachiocrural myoclonia that had appeared the day before, beginning in the left upper extremity. The parents were first cousins. EEG showed a generalized tracing of epileptogenic activity with slow punctiform waves that clearly predominated in the right cerebral hemisphere. Spinal fluid was normal. There was no hypoglycemia. Blood magnesium, calcium, phosphorus, and phosphatase levels were normal. X-ray examination of the skeleton showed generalized homogeneous increase in the density of bone affecting the entire skeleton, with complete disappearance of medullary canals in the long bones and no spongy structure in any bone, an extreme example of "marble bone" disease. Some of the long tubular bones such as the humerus, radius, and tibia showed incomplete metaphyseal infundibulization, the shape resembling that of a bottle. The diagnosis was Albers-Schonberg disease. Anticonvulsant treatment was instituted, and the child was discharged with that diagnosis 10 days later. An EEG at the time showed high, slow polymorphous waves in opposing phases over a large segment of the right temporoparietal region. Seven days later she was readmitted with an acute respiratory disease diagnosed as bacterial pneumonia, of which she died 3 days later.

Histopathologic Examination. Figure 367 represents the midportion of a rib. Abnormally large numbers of trabeculae, as well as increased thickness of each, produce a reduction in the medullary space. There is very little hematopoietic tissue. The bony trabeculae, for the most part, show a residual cartilaginous matrix normal for the age of the child. Mineralization is scanty, and the lines of apposition are poorly visualized, while there is still a considerable amount of osteoid (H & E, 60 ×).

Figure 368 represents the image obtained by means of fluorescence with acridine orange stain. The cartilaginous matrix stands out because of its violet color, and the scanty zone of calcification takes on a golden yellow hue. The blue bands represent nonmineralized osteoid (375 ×).

At autopsy, a granulocytic pneumonia was discovered with bronchitis and bronchiolitis and foci of hematopoiesis in the liver and spleen.

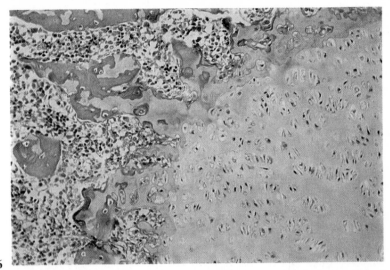

366

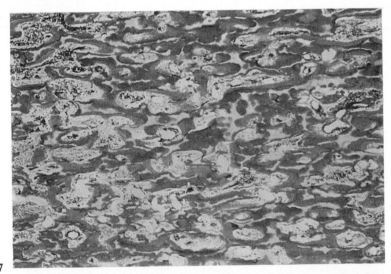

367

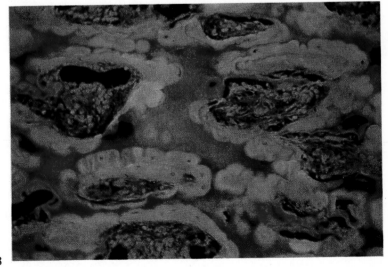

368

Congenital Tumors*

369
BENIGN HEMANGIOENDOTHELIOMA

Female weighing 3,400 gm. Gestational age, 38 weeks. Admitted at 4 days of life with a mass in the left shoulder. Examination showed a movable soft tumor with an irregular wine-red surface that was diagnosed as hemangioma. Following surgical resection of the mass, the child was discharged at 14 days of age.

Histopathologic Examination. Microscopically this is a poorly defined hamartoma made up of small newly formed capillaries with poorly defined or nonexistent lumina lined by regular endothelial cells without signs of atypia, the solid angioblastic cellular component predominating (H & E, 375 ×).

370
CAVERNOUS HEMANGIOMA

Male weighing 3,400 gm. Gestational age, 38 weeks. Admitted at 8 days of life because of a mass in the left shoulder, which had been increasing in size progressively. Physical examination showed a localized swelling the size of a hen's egg, soft, fluctuant, and with a light wine-red color, located over the scapulo-humeral joint. X-ray showed calcification within the tumor mass. The remainder of the physical examination was normal. The mass was removed surgically, and the child was released 8 days later.

Histopathologic Examination. The tumor was located in the subcutaneous tissue. It was soft and deep red. Microscopically, it is made up partly of a large number of blood vessels of varying caliber and partly of cavernous dilated spaces, all of them filled with red blood cells. The walls of the vessels are delicate, with an endothelial lining overlying a relatively thin band of connective tissue (H & E, 187.5 ×).

371
LYMPHANGIOMA

Male weighing 3,700 gm. Gestational age, 40 weeks. Admitted 20 days after birth because of a mass on the dorsum of the right hand that involved the dorsal aspect of the thumb. Clinically, it was considered to be a lymphangioma. The mass was soft and bluish-white. It was removed surgically.

Histopathologic Examination. The mass is made up of numerous lymphatics, many of them greatly dilated and containing homogeneous eosinophilic material in their lumina. The walls of the vessels are thin, and each is lined by a single layer of endothelial cells (H & E, 187.5 ×).

372
CYSTIC HYGROMA OF THE NECK (LYMPHANGIOMA)

Male weighing 3,600 gm. Gestational age, 38 weeks. Admitted 2 days after delivery because of a large mass in the cervical region.

Examination showed a mass in the left cervical region, large, soft, and adherent to both the deeper and the superficial tissues. The remainder of the examination was normal. An x-ray was unrevealing. The mass was removed surgically, and the child was discharged 10 days later.

Histopathologic Examination. The tumor was made up of large cystic cavities filled with clear fluid. Figure 372 shows two wide lymphatic lumina with delicate endothelial lining. The stroma is made up of loose connective tissue with mild round cell infiltration (H & E, 375 ×).

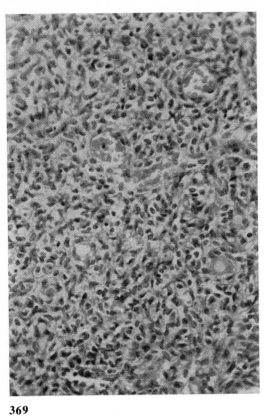

369

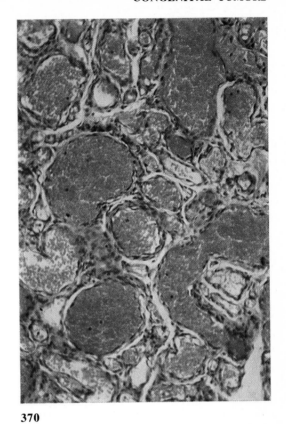

370

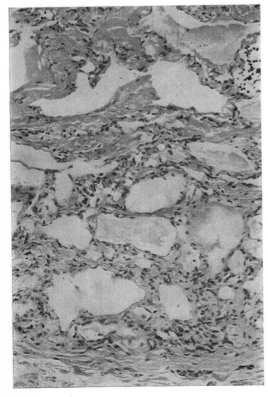

371

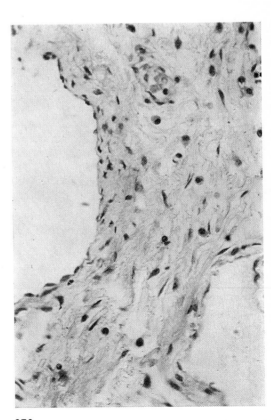

372

373/374
SACRAL TERATOMA

Female weighing 3,350 gm. Gestational age, 38 weeks. Delivery by cesarean section. Admitted at 2 hours of life because of a large tumor mass in the sacrococcygeal region.

Examination disclosed no other pathologic change. Clinically, the tumor was considered to be a sacrococcygeal teratoma. Surgical resection was accomplished, and the child was released 12 days after admission.

Histopathologic Examination. Grossly the tumor was solid, weighing 210 gm. Microscopically, it was composed of various well-differentiated tissues derived from the three blastodermic layers.

Figure 373 shows a cavity lined by columnar epithelium and ensheathed in layered smooth muscle (upper left corner); a plaque of hyaline cartilage appears near the center of the photograph (H & E, 375 ×).

Figure 374 shows another field made up of glial tissue (H & E, 375 ×).

375
EMBRYONAL RHABDOMYOSARCOMA

Male weighing 3,200 gm. Gestational age, 38 weeks. Admitted 5 days after birth with low intestinal obstruction. Aganglionic megacolon was diagnosed by x-ray and confirmed by frozen section.

Twelve days later a mass began to develop on the left side of the abdominal wall. It grew rapidly until it reached the size of a pigeon's egg. It was located subcutaneously and did not adhere to the skin. It was attached to muscle and was soft. The skin covering the mass was dark. Rapid growth led to the suspicion that the tumor was malignant, and a biopsy was performed.

Histopathologic Examination. Microscopically, this is a markedly cellular mass made up of poorly differentiated cells with irregular nuclei. There are a few rhabdomyoblasts, each in the shape of a tennis racquet, with eosinophilic cytoplasm. Figure 375 represents a pleomorphic and rather myxoid area (H & E, 375 ×).

376
CHORIOCARCINOMA

Male weighing, 3,200 gm. Gestational age, 38 weeks. Admitted 6 days after birth because of a left retroauricular mass. On admission his general condition was good. There was a mass located behind the left ear that was said to have grown rapidly in the preceding 3 days and that suggested an angioma.

Physical examination was normal, and there were no other changes. The lesion was excised. Later, in view of the malignant character of the neoplasm and because of the possibility that the excised tumor could be metastatic from a primary tumor located elsewhere, a more thorough, general physical examination was carried out, but did not reveal any primary tumor. The child was discharged at the request of the parents. He died at home at 1 month of age.

Histopathologic Examination. The dermis is invaded by irregular syncytiotrophoblastic cells that are markedly atypical, together with cytotrophoblastic nests, vascular clefts, and extensive hemorrhagic necrotic areas. Figure 376 represents one edge of the tumor (H & E, 187.5 ×).

OTHER TUMORS OBSERVED IN INFANTS UP TO 30 DAYS OF AGE CAN BE SEEN IN:

Figure 132/133. Rhabdomyoma of the heart.
Figure 147/148/149. Giant teratoma of the brain.
Figure 170. Nodule of undifferentiated renal blastema.
Figure 188/189/190/191. Renal nephroblastomatosis.
Figure 204. Congenital epulis.
Figure 209. Hemagioma of the parotid.
Figure 225. Metastatic neuroblastoma in the pancreas.
Figure 294. Cavernous hemagioma of the liver.
Figure 295. Mesenchymal hamartoma of the liver.
Figure 296/297. Massive invasion of liver by congenital neuroblastoma.
Figure 319. Neuroblastoma.

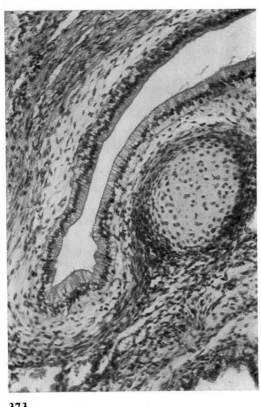

373

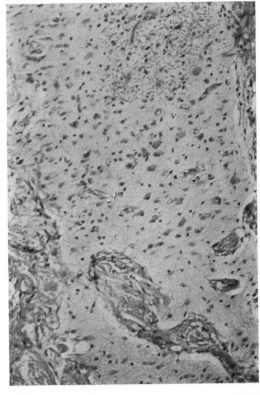

374

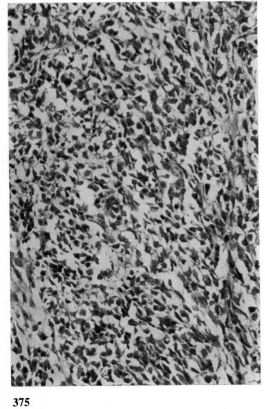

375

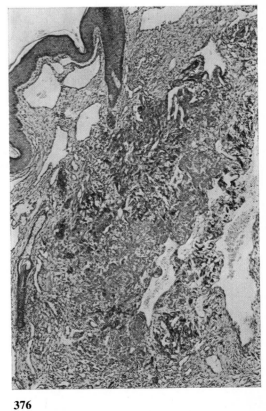

376

Index

Page numbers in *italics* refer to illustrations.

INDEX